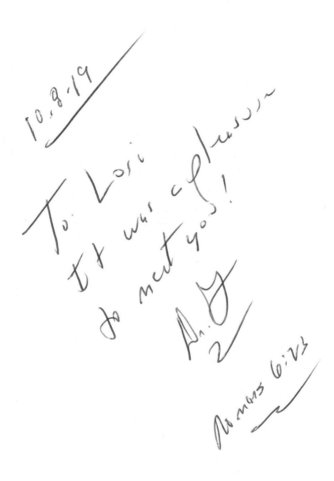

10.8.19

To: Lori
It was a pleasure
to meet you!

A.G.

Romans 6:23

D1378327

You Never Know How

Far-Reaching

Something You

Think, Say, or Do

TODAY

Will Affect

The Lives of Millions

TOMORROW.

-B.J. Palmer-
Developer of Chiropractic

Don't Get the Screws Put to You!

7 Steps to Prevent the Knife

Written by

Dr. Stephen L. Graham,
Back Pain Professor

Foreword by

David A. Weber, M.D.,
Harvard Medical

Illustrated by

Kaylee Cheser

Disclaimer and Terms of Use: Your reliance upon information and content obtained by you through this publication is solely at your own risk. The author assumes no liability or responsibility for damage or injury to you, other persons, or property arising from use of any product, information, idea, or instruction contained in the content provided to you through this book.

TABLE OF CONTENTS

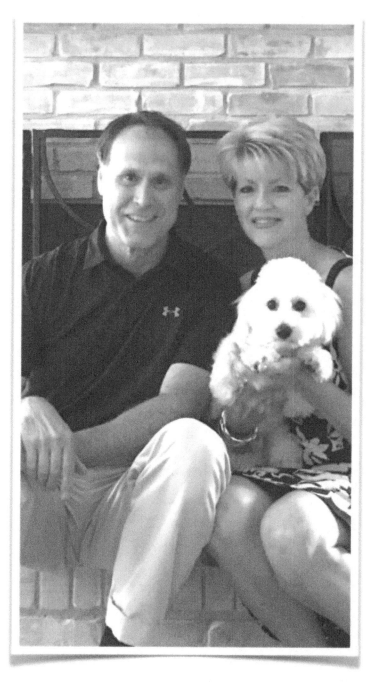

I dedicate this book to my wife, Donna. I stayed in the basement many a day and night working on this book, while she took care of our home and our little Samson.

Acknowledgements:

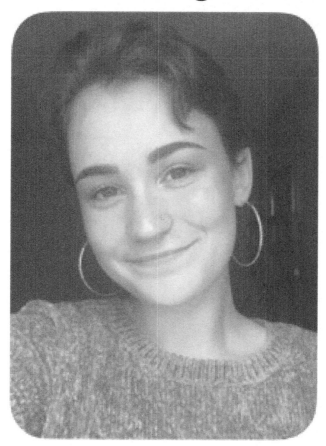

Kaylee Cheser

- *Lead Illustrator*
- *Front Cover Artist*

Contributing Illustrators:

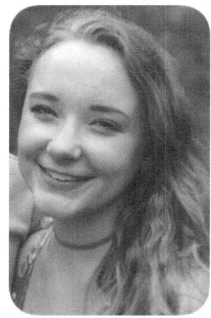

Emily Parker

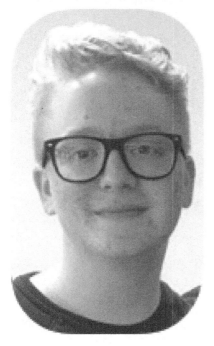

Coby Young

Back cover photography: Tara Haskins

FOREWORD

Back pain is a very difficult condition to get a handle on, even for this doctor who has specialized in this one area of the spine for many years. With multi-million-dollar MRI tubes and endless testing strategies, overcoming and correcting back pain can be like chasing the wind. That is why back pain is a $100,000,000,000 ($100 billion) a year epidemic.

After over twenty years of working in this field, I am now as convinced as Dr. Graham is, that the real way to combat back pain is with prevention. Preventive care is far better than ingesting pain pills, getting injections, or even worse going under the knife. More times than not, surgery or surgeries, only leads to a life of chronic pain, disability, and finally a loss of interest in living.

As an interventional spine specialist, I have heard many different ideas on how to prevent back pain. However, the seven ways Dr. Graham has outlined in his book, I believe to be spot on. He has laid out each principle with great stories, x-rays and even comprehensive case studies. However, the real genius of the book lays in the fact that he has made it easy to understand for anyone. I could easily deduce that it was written over a long period because of how well each chapter was thought out.

I especially liked how he tells an interesting story to introduce each chapter in a self-deprecating manner. I found *Aligning and Decompressing the Spine: The Final Step* and *It's the Core* to be very compelling chapters. I have to say though, I especially enjoyed the Bonus Materials; *10 Most "Jacked Up" Spines of the Year!* and *Holy Titanium.*

When Dr. G and I had dinner a few months ago, he told me for the last two years he had been writing a book. He said he was now putting the finishing touches on it and asked me if I would write his

xv

foreword. I told him not only that I would, but how honored I was that he asked me to do it.

It did not surprise me at all that he wrote this book because of his commitment level to his profession and his patients. There is hardly a week that goes by that I don't get a text from him that reads, 'I know you are busy and I hate to bother you, but what do you think of this x-ray?'

Dr. Graham is dedicated, he is compassionate, and he is pretty humorous. I believe all these qualities is what makes him the great chiropractor I know him to be. However, after reading this book, I now can say, I know him to be a pretty good author, also.

In conclusion, I asked Dr. Graham that same evening at dinner, what compelled him to write a book on back pain. He told me he wanted to give something tangible to his patients that would help them to take more ownership with the health of their back. After reading this, I will take it a step further by adding that this is not only a handbook for people with back pain, but more importantly it is for the bigger population of people, who have not yet suffered with back pain.

According to the United States Census Bureau there are 126.22 million households in the United States as of 2017. If each household followed the seven steps outlined in Dr. Graham's handbook, it would probably eliminate 80% of the back surgeries across the United States. Talk about moving the total healthcare bill needle!

Thank you again Dr. G. for letting me be a part of your book, it was truly an honor!

David A. Weber, M.D.
Interventional Pain Specialist
Board Certified in Anesthesia and Pain Management
Fellowship Trained in Pain Medicine,
Massachusetts General Hospital-Harvard University

PREFACE

God's Strange Arithmetic

Weeping may tarry for the night,
but joy comes with the morning.
                              -Psalms 30:5

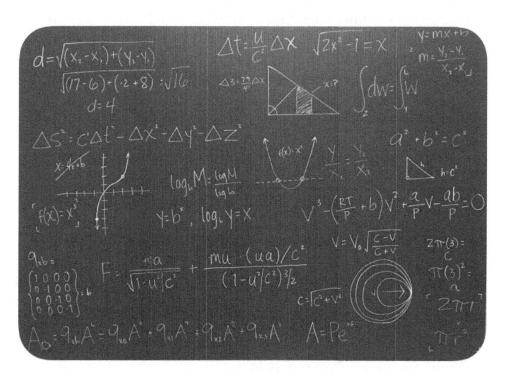

"...what could I have done to prevent this?"

A few years ago, I was sitting across the table from an executive that managed a large company in Louisville. He was in his late fifties and suffering with back pain and leg pain so severe, that he could barely sit through our consultation. One thing that I will never forget was the fear I saw in his eyes because of the probability that he may be facing fusion surgery.

His head was down during most of my questioning. At one point toward the end of our consultation, he raised his head and looked me square in the eyes, as if he had already given in to the idea of surgery, and he said to me, "Dr. Graham, as I was staring at the top of the MRI tube, I thought 'what could I have done to prevent this?"

I stared at him in silence for a few seconds, because I didn't think he was really looking for an answer to his question, but more for a listening ear.

His rhetorical question though, did get me thinking, just what was the answer? This man's query that morning, turned out to be the genesis of this book.

I wanted to put in writing an answer to my patient's query.

So, for the past two years I have painstakingly, formulated a simple guide that will not only help my patients through their road to recovery, but will also help to prevent the average person from ever experiencing back pain.

I believe, that had this gentleman had a copy of this book, ten years earlier, he would not have ever been on the inside of an MRI tube, facing fusion surgery and wondering how on earth he ever got there!

80-20

Although two years was spent on this book, the dots really connect back to a hot Friday afternoon, in the summer of 1980.

At the end of my junior year at Bellarmine College, I interviewed for a summer banking job at a local credit union. I must have made a pretty good impression because they hired me right on the spot. After just six weeks of work, my supervisor asked me to come to her office. I actually thought she was going to talk to me about a raise, but instead, she fired me!

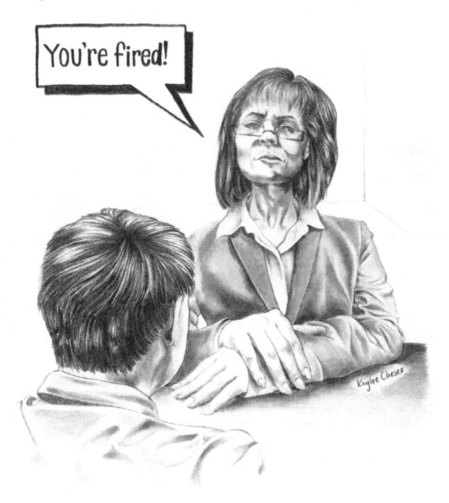

I remember like it was yesterday how embarrassed and humiliated I was when I walked out the door.

By the time I got home, I felt even more embarrassed. So much so, that I was 80-20 in favor of me not telling my parents. The percentages played out and for the next seven weeks before I went back to school; I continued to get up at the same time, suit up, and play "banker". My parents never did find out their son got fired that summer, or for that matter, ever!

Since I had just started taking an evening accelerated cost accounting class at Bellarmine College, I just hung out there all day studying. The last thing I needed to do was fail, then for sure I would have been, unquestionably, the biggest loser in the summer of '80!

I could not have had better parents!

I just couldn't bear to tell them that their son got fired after only 6 weeks on the job!

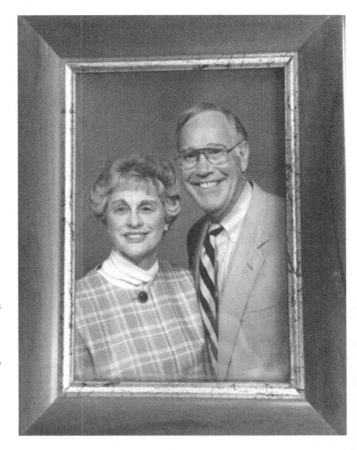

A Day that Changed it All

I could only study so much for accounting, so to kill some time I went to the gym on campus and worked out. So, there on a Thursday afternoon, I was in a hurry and did not warm up first. This is a no-no especially with doing squats!

I rested the bar across my shoulders, loaded with 150 pounds. As I looked in the mirror in anticipation of my first rep, I slowly bent my knees, and in the matter of a split second, I heard a loud pop in my lower back. I immediately dropped the weights and knew right then and there, I had jacked-up up a perfectly healthy back!

To make a long story short, my back stayed screwed up for the next two plus years and was not showing any signs of getting better. I was graduating in accounting and studying for my CPA exam and even still, some thirty-seven years later, I can still recall how painful those 28 months were.

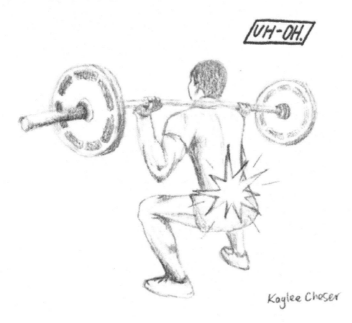

Kaylee Choser

I had just jacked-up a perfectly healthy back!

These are 6 rejection letters I received...

I have held on to these letters, all these years, as a reminder to me that...

...from all 6 National Accounting firms that I interviewed with my senior year.

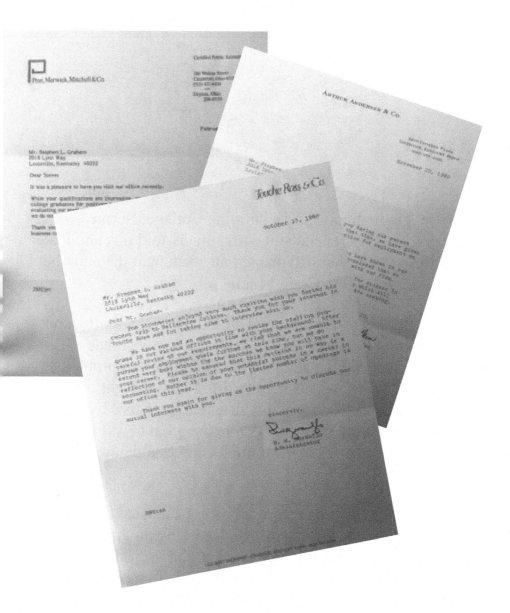

...disappointments and defeats are part of life, but they are only temporal.

A Chiropractor Saves my Back!

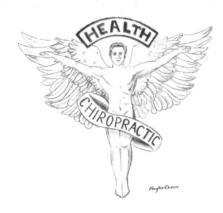

After graduating from Bellarmine College, Bernie Lubbers, my great friend since first grade, told me, about a new chiropractor that had opened an account at the bank he was working for, Dr. Craig Mueller.

I went to his office later that week. After examining and taking two x-rays of my spine, he explained what had happened. He said the weight of the barbells had probably misaligned my spine causing my disc to bulge right into my sciatic nerve. He said he could un-pinch my nerve by re-aligning my spine. Then he told me the great news! He said that he thought he could have me feeling brand new in 6-12 weeks.

After four weeks of getting my spine adjusted back into alignment, my leg pain, that I had for going on three years, disappeared. It was not long after that, that my back was normal again. It was almost inconceivable to me, how my problem was fixed without any drugs, needles, or surgery, but just with someone's bare hands moving my spine back in the proper alignment. I thought it to be nothing short of a miracle.

Off to Chiropractic School

I was ecstatic, not only because my pain was gone, but I knew at this point, I wanted to go to chiropractic school to become a chiropractor.

At that time, there were just sixteen chiropractic schools in the United States. After researching the different schools, I decided on Logan College in St. Louis, mainly because it was rated as one of the top schools in the nation, and it was only three hundred miles from Louisville. In 1985, I headed out for Missouri to attend Logan College of Chiropractic!

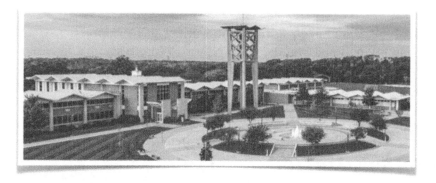

Logan Chiropractic College used to be a seminary, but due to the declining interest of men joining the Priesthood, they closed the doors and Logan purchased the property.

Logan was included in MSNBC's 2007 list of "America's Most Beautiful College Campuses".

My brother David, was a young Pathologist at the time. He told me Logan was very similar to University of Louisville medical school, as we were studying the same courses and even books that he did, like anatomy, physiology, histology, pathology, cell biology, biochemistry, etc. However, when it came to treatment, it is different, in that medical students learned about drugs and surgery, whereas we learned how to achieve better health by taking stress off the nervous system, by aligning the spine.

My first semester courses at Logan Chiropractic College (1986).

I have to admit I was a little intimidated by this course load!

Doctor of Chiropractic Degree Curriculum
Schedule Effective January 1984

Trimester I

Course No.	Title	Average Clock Hours per Week			Trimester Clock Hours
		Lect.	Lab.	Credit	
1111	Logan Principles & Philosophy of Body Mechanics I	2	0	2	30
1141	Spinal Analysis I	2	1	2.5	45
1311	Chiropractic Philosophy	3	0	3	45
1411	Gross Anatomy I	4	5	6.5	135
1421	Histology	3	2	4	75
1431	Orthopedy	4	0	4	60
1511	Cell Biology	2	0	2	30
1551	Scientific Etymology	3	0	3	45
1811	Normal X-Ray	1	0	1	15
		24	8	28.0	480

In 1989, I graduated from Logan College of Chiropractic. After passing my national boards, in March of 1990, I became a licensed Chiropractor in the Commonwealth of Kentucky. I opened Graham Chiropractic Center on May 1, 1990, and have been here ever since!

Me with my brother, David.

He is the "real doctor" in our family.

Just like I did growing up, I can still take him in ping-pong!

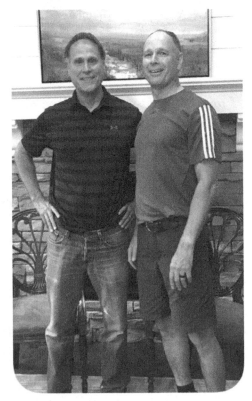

In the x-ray lab, analyzing and marking x-rays.

Good thing I enjoy geometry!

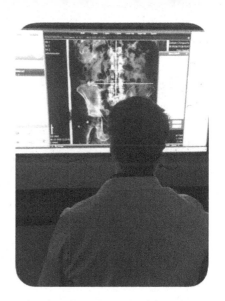

Engineering more than Doctoring

I have always thought of myself to be more of an engineer than a doctor, because I analyze the abnormal stresses that are put on the vertebral column. When the spine becomes abnormally stressed, the discs, which are nestled between the vertebrae, begin to degenerate (1), causing a whole host of problems, the main one being pain and discomfort. My job is to re-align the spine, to take the stresses and strains off the disc, and to give the body a chance to heal.

On my wall, at the entrance to my office, I have a quote by Hippocrates, the Father of Medicine. It reads:

"Look well to the spine for the cause of disease."

Sounds pretty much like a chiropractor to me!

Magical Numbers

There are few defining moments in everyone's life. At the time, it is impossible to know if, what appears to be an insignificant event, will be defining or just some random thing that had no consequence for the good or for the bad. The only way to know for sure, is if the dots connect to something great in the future.

If it were not for me getting fired from that credit union job, I probably would have never enrolled in chiropractic school and could not have experienced, "God's Strange Arithmetic."

- Since becoming a chiropractor, my life has been *doubly* enriched, because I continue waking up every morning doing something I love doing.
- I probably never would have met my wife, Donna, who is at least *three* times better than anyone else that I could ever have married!
- And I believe that this book will end up touching *thousands* of lives, that otherwise, I would never have been able to touch!

So, the dots did connect, and what had appeared to have been a very bad Friday afternoon that I wanted to forget about, was actually just God preparing my table for some strange arithmetic, that would come later.

My hope for you, is when your back becomes strong and pain free, that your dots connect back to this book!

Stephen h. Graham
— D.C. —

INTRODUCTION

It's All Screwed Up!

There is a way that appears right,
but in the end it leads to destruction.

-Proverbs 14:12

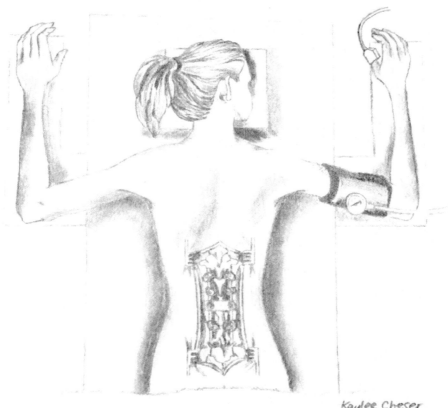

Kaylee Cheser

One evening while I was serving my internship at the Montgomery Health Center, I was assigned a patient that came into our clinic with severe back pain. During the consultation, this man of about 45 years, told me that he underwent fusion surgery two years earlier. As a young intern, I eagerly marked this on his chart without really understanding the potential ramifications of this type of surgery.

Following my examination, I took two x-rays of his lumbar spine (low back). Within a few short minutes, the x-ray tech slapped up both films on the view box, as if they were just some irrelevant sticky notes. As I got closer to the x-rays, I could not help but stare in amazement at the metallic shimmer of four metal screws that had been drilled right through this man's spinal bones.

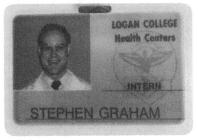

I was so proud to start my internship at Montgomery Clinic.

It felt like such a long road, and I finally had made it!

That marked the very first time that I actually got that close and upfront to a real spinal fusion. This x-ray had a life of its own, as if it were breathing. This man lived in a very nice neighborhood, just down the street from Logan's clinic. He was a husband, a dad, and he was probably someone's brother and uncle. This was not just some x-ray out of a text book that I had seen countless times before. This was a real person!

That night at the clinic in 1988, I was introduced to spinal fusions. It was just two years later, in 1990, when I began my chiropractic practice, that I got a real taste for the number of people who had these types of surgeries. More amazing though, than the number that were performed, were the number of these that did not work, leaving these poor people with scars and metal permanently lodged in their back.

Even today, in 2018, I hear the same words being strung together by these fusion recipients, that I heard 28 years ago, "Dr. Graham, I will never, ever have another surgery. I don't care how much my back hurts."

"...I kept thinking the next one would work."

A patient of mine, Mr. B, made a 100-mile round trip to my clinic from Fort Knox in Kentucky, because he had unrelenting back pain. As he was lying face down on the examination table, he said, "Dr. Graham, it hurts right along that long scar I have in my back." It was a long, thick unsightly incision, which almost looked like a blending of scars.

Mr. B had 14 back surgeries!

I replied with, "Mr. B, exactly how many surgeries am I looking at here?" It was a shocker to hear him say, fourteen!

I said "fourteen?"

He repeated, "Yes, fourteen". He then went on to say, "Dr. Graham for the past 44 years I have been living in pain, ever since I fell off of a deer stand and landed on my back. I have had surgery after surgery and I kept thinking that the next one would work."

Although, I have never seen any other patients that have had fourteen surgeries, I have treated patients that have had upwards of five. It is very common in my practice to treat people who have had two and three back surgeries. Most of them tell me the same thing: I would never, ever go under the knife again.

Some patients that have never had surgery tell me that their brother, mom, dad, or friend had surgery or multiple operations and their back still hurts. Now, I am not so naïve to think that none of these work, because I do hear plenty of times that low back surgery has relieved people of their pain. In fact, I have referred a number of patients, through my 27 years of service, out for surgery. A number of them worked out well, and they continued to live healthier lives.

3

Many surgeons save operating on the back as a last resort. Some have even told my patients to stay away from back surgery, unless absolutely nothing else has worked, meaning medicine, injections, physical therapy, chiropractic care, etc. You get the idea.

As I stared in disbelief in 1988, at those 4 shiny screws on that view box, I am sure the question crossed my mind of whether or not, in 25 years, this type of surgery would phase out. Let me tell you, it is far from extinct!

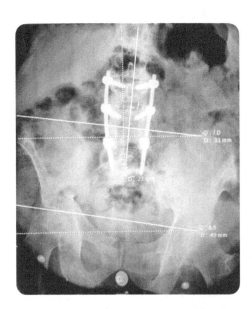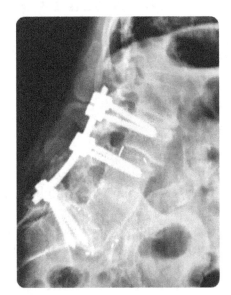

Mr. B's low back in 2017.

474% vs 16%, What the Hay???

Over a 15-year period between 1996 and 2011, the number of spinal fusion surgeries had risen from 98,000 to 465,000. That is more than a fourfold increase. (1)

I did some quick "back of the napkin math" to see what the population increase was between 1996 and 2011 (269M to 311M) and it came to 16% growth (2)!

Nothing like the old school way to arrive at a 15.6% increase.

Who needs an iPhone!

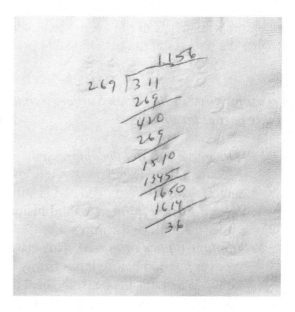

So, what's with the 474% increase, when the population grew only 16% in this period?

Some experts say that it is the aging population, while some stretch it even further, saying it is the rising demand for an active lifestyle among older people (3). For me, I am just not sure.

Failed Back Surgery Syndrome

Failed Back Surgery Syndrome is a very generalized term that is often used to describe the condition of patients who have not had a successful result with back surgery. Research studies show that out of all the back surgeries performed, 22% of recipients needed a second procedure (4). I would say that at least one in five of my patients, roughly 20%, that have had back surgery, had a repeat surgery on the same area.

I don't know the exact percentages, but I would estimate that easily, more than half of the surgical cases that I am aware of, did not provide the pain relief the patient had hoped for.

9 reasons why "Failed Back Surgery Syndrome" is so prevalent (not in any particular order) (5).

1. *The nerve was not decompressed.* Sometimes this occurs because a bone fragment was left, or some herniated disc material was not removed and is still pressing on the nerve.
2. *Spinal Fusion failure.* A solid fusion never occurred with either the graft or the implant.
3. *Implant slipped or moved.* This usually occurs during the recovery period before it has firmly attached to the spinal bone. When this happens, the heal may be less effective or not effective at all. Or yet, it could damage the nerve tissue and make the condition worse.
4. *Scar tissue formation.* These fibrous adhesions are part of the healing process, but they can also bind around a nerve root.
5. *Nerve damage.* In rare cases, nerve damage occurs and can cause chronic pain and weakness.
6. *An incorrect diagnosis.*
7. *Performing the surgery at an incorrect level.*
8. Fusion surgery that *transfers problems to another level of the spine*, causing a new level of degeneration and pain. This typically occurs more with multi-level fusions. This is known as adjacent segment disease.
9. And of course, if the *surgery is unnecessary.*

8 Adjacent Segment Disease

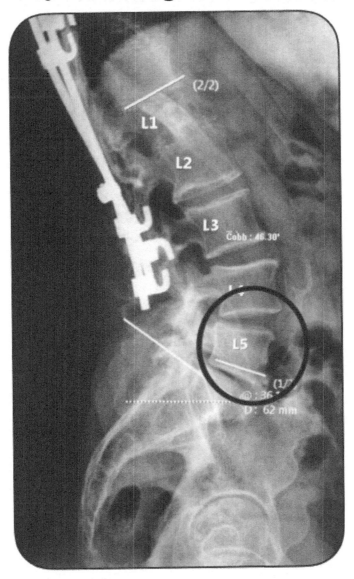

The adjacent levels tend to degenerate at an accelerated rate because of the increased load and stress.

Risks involved with surgery!

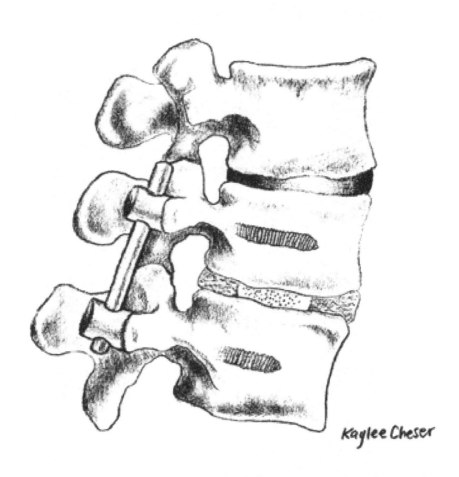

Kaylee Cheser

Recently, Keith, a very pleasant 51-year-old, entered our office. He was very distraught from the severe left leg pain he was experiencing. His MRI revealed a moderately degenerated disc, with a disc bulge measuring 6mm at L5-S1. This bulge was pressing directly on the sciatic nerve.

This is Keith's pain pattern

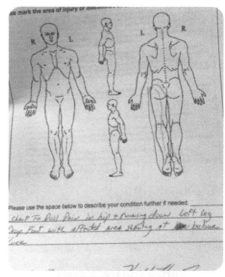

This is his MRI.

You can easily see the bulge that is causing his leg pain.

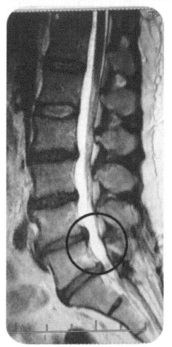

Keith said that he was considering surgery and asked me about the risks associated with this.

I face this question often as to whether or not someone should follow through with surgery. I told Keith what I tell everyone else, which is: there are many risks associated with back surgery, seven of the main ones being (6).

1. Anesthesia

2. Infection

3. Blood loss

4. Nerve injury

5. Lack of a solid fusion

6. Complications such as pneumonia, heart attack, stroke, and blood clots

7. Increased pain

There are only a few situations where I believe surgery is absolutely necessary, one being extreme weakness in the leg muscles and the other being a *loss of bowel or bladder control.*

Occasionally, patients with these findings may find their way to my office for help. Years ago, while consulting with a patient, he brought to my attention, that he had lost control of his bowel and bladder. I stopped the consultation and sent him to the hospital for emergency surgery. This instance has happened only once in my 27-year career.

Facts About Back Pain *(7)*

- *8 out of 10 will experience back problems at some point in their life.*

- *Back problems are more common in women (30.2) than men (26.4).*

- *The majority of back pain comes from desk workers: 54%*

- *More than one in three adults say back pain impacts their everyday activities, including sleep.*

- *$50,000,000,000 of treatments in 2016.*

- *$100,000,000,000 of indirect costs in 2016.*

To put this in perspective, $100 billion would buy:

-200 million iPads (enough for every U.S. school and college student).

-33.3 billion Starbucks caffe lattes

-3600 islands worth $25 million each, like Dark Island, Vermont. (8)

There was more spent on back pain in 2016 ($100 billion), than the following companies collected in revenues in 2017, according to Forbes:

- ✓ *Wells Fargo $97.7B*
- ✓ *Boeing   93.3*
- ✓ *Phillips 66   91.6*
- ✓ *Anthem   90.0*
- ✓ *Microsoft   89.9*

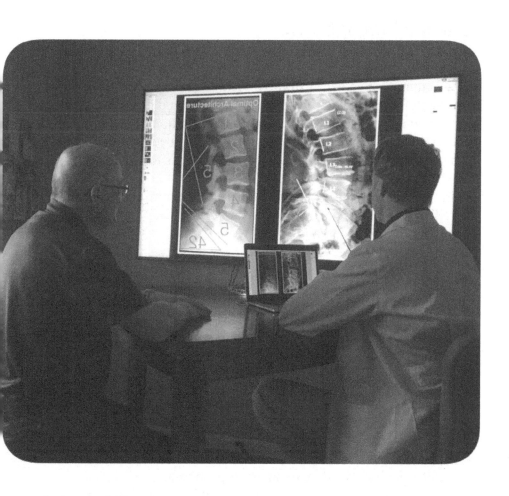

Me with a patient reviewing his low back case.

I really enjoy this profession because I have met so many nice people including Marvin, who is in this picture with me.

One final thought......

Most of us are familiar with the Farmers Insurance theme, "We know a thing or two because we've seen a thing or two!" Well, from my twenty-seven years of being a chiropractor and probably having performed more than 12,000 back pain consultations, examinations and x-rays, I have gotten to learn a thing or two because I have seen a thing or two. In fact, I have seen about all there is to see!

In this handbook, I have laid out the seven most important ingredients to having a healthy back based on these 12,000 patients I have talked to, gotten to know, and treated.

- I have seen many collapsing arches that I corrected with a "3-Arch" Orthotic, only to see both their back and knee issues clear up. Some of these same patients had even been scheduled for surgery.

- I have seen my patient's back pain evaporate after prescribing core exercises.

- I have seen patients get on a walking program and have seen both their weight and back pain disappear.

- I have instructed them on better posture and given many prescriptions for stand-up desks and have witnessed their chronic back pain fall by the wayside.

- I have consulted with patients about mattress sag or having too many springs in their bed. I have recommended the best mattress to sleep on, only to see their back get better.

- And I have adjusted thousands of patient's spines where they told me it was nothing short of a miracle when their back pain, that they have had for years, disappeared sometimes in a matter of months, weeks or even days!

Hopefully by following your handbook, you can one day launch a healthier path and stop taking:

Ibuprofen and Tylenol that tax your liver and kidneys (9,10),

prescription drugs, the 4th leading cause of death in the United States (11) whose side effects are often far worse than your back pain,

steroid injections that soften your bones and cause compression fractures (12),

and that you never have to face...

...having the screws put to you!

THE BEGINNINGS

Our Framework

"The doctor of the future will give no medicine but will interest his patients in the care of the human frame (spine), in diet, and the prevention of disease"

-Thomas A. Edison

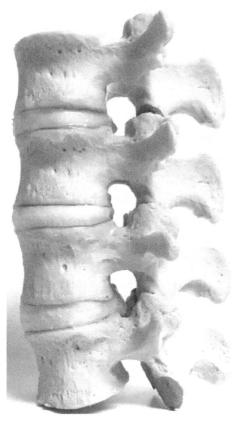

Spinal Anatomy for Dummies

1969 was a great year for me! The New York Jets, with Joe Namath, defeated Johnny Unitus and the Baltimore Colts in the Super Bowl III. That same year, I watched the very first man to land on the moon on our black and white 19" Zenith television. As if that was not already enough, in that same year, Pope Paul VI issued an updated version of the Catholic mass that dropped the Latin (1)! So, my slumbering at church was literally cut in half overnight!

Now, fast forward 16 years. I was in Chiropractic school sitting in anatomy class, but it felt like I was back in a 1968 St. Albert's Latin service. Because most of the anatomy language is derived from Latin roots, there was a sense of familiarity when learning parts of the body, like the muscle, Latissimus Dorsi.

Dr. Ellis, my anatomy instructor, despite all the Latin, was able to make anatomy fun, through things like mnemonics. Anatomy for dummies if you will. An example of this was, "C3-4-5 keeps the diaphragm alive" (referring to the nerves that control the diaphragm)! Goofy stuff, but it worked for me. It was no wonder that Dr. Ellis was awarded teacher of the year multiple times!

So, my goal with this chapter is to make anatomy fun, the Ellis way!

Spinal Anatomy for Dummies

The spine is made of 24 bones with 23 discs sandwiched in between each vertebra (2).

Spinal Cord

4th vertebrae in the lower back

Disc

The nerve exits between the two vertebrae

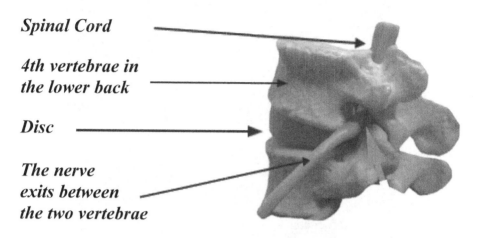

If the disc is not neglected, it will eliminate the majority of back pain in the United States of America!

Our spine is made of a strong encasement of bones that act to protect the most important system in the body, the central nervous system. This is made up of the brain and the spinal cord (3). That way, if we have a slip or fall on ice or down the steps, our spinal cord will be well guarded.

My brother, Jeff, a very sharp engineer in his own right, who also is known to be sometimes on the clumsy side, had a tough fall a few years ago. He was clipping a branch in his tree and fell hitting the ground hard in his front yard. Good thing for him, because of the sturdy, hard bones our spine has, they did not fracture, but he did manage to break his arm.

I can remember telling him after his spill that if he was going to fall, at least do it somewhere that will pay the bill, like a Burger King or Kmart (just kidding of course)!

This is the arm he broke...oops!

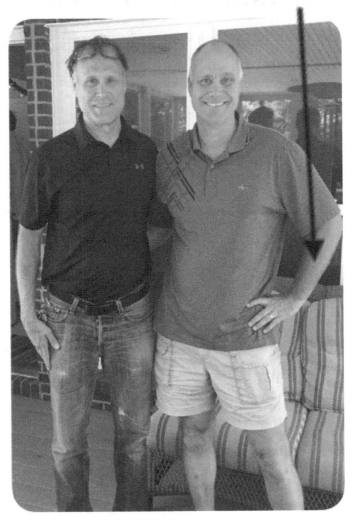

My brother Jeff and me at his son, Alex's graduation party.

Alex will be attending my Alma Mater, Bellarmine University, to study biology. His plan is to enroll in medical school.

Jeff, like my brother David, is quite the biker!

It's the Disc!

During my 27 years of working with back pain, in my opinion, most people's backs deteriorates because their disc is going bad, and..

......since the disc is the key to having a healthy back, I am devoting the rest of this chapter to its anatomy.

The word disc is tossed around a lot in the chiropractic and medical profession, especially in x-ray and MRI (Magnetic Resonance Imaging) reports. I even have to watch myself, because sometimes I can get numb to the fact that Joe Public does not really know what a disc is, or for that matter, what it does.

There are twenty-three discs in our spine. The discs in the lower back are about ½ inch thick, while the other discs in the neck and mid back are closer to 1/4 of an inch (4). They are made of a hard rubber material called an annulus, with a jelly-like material in the middle, called the nucleus pulposus (5).

normal

The disc begins losing its automatic blood supply after the age of 5.

After that, it relies on healthy spinal bones to pump the blood through, to keep them well hydrated.

This is why good alignment is important.

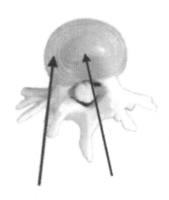

annulus   *nucleus*

There are three main functions of the disc (6).

1. Gives flexibility to the spine.
2. Gives shock absorption to the spine.
3. Acts as a spacer, to make for a larger opening for the nerve to pass through

The disc provides:

flexibility

shock absorption

acts as a spacer, to make a larger opening for the nerves to pass through

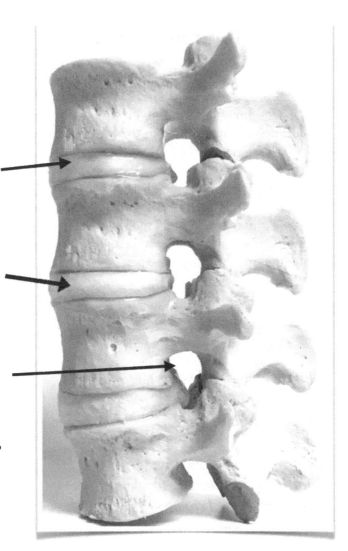

As an example of the first two (flexibility and shock absorption), think of Simone Biles, the gold medal winning gymnast in the 2016 Summer Olympics. Remember how she was able to bend, twist, and then land from ten feet in the air, directly on to her feet? Nourished, thick discs made it possible for her to do that! If she had a worn-out disc in her back, there's a high likelihood, that she would have had a compression fracture or two, from all of the forces going throughout her spine on her ten-foot landing.

Normal Disc

The best way to evaluate a disc is by an MRI. Unlike an x-ray, which only shows if the disc is thick or thin, the MRI can reveal if the disc is hydrated, desiccated (dehydrated), degenerated, bulging, or herniated.

This is an MRI showing healthy discs.

You can see that the discs are white. This means that they are full of water, or hydrated.

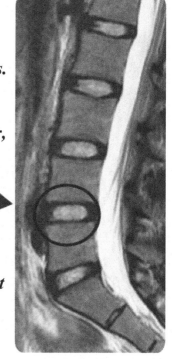

Hydration is good, because when the disc is hydrated it is strong and the jelly material is in the middle, and not as likely to bulge or herniate.

A healthy disc is made up of 70-80% water (7). On an MRI, if the disc is properly hydrated it will look white (see previous page). The jelly material (ball bearing) will usually be in the middle. In addition, well hydrated discs are thicker, thus providing a larger opening for the spinal nerve. Lastly, a hydrated disc is a better shock absorber, allowing the spine to better handle activities, like running and jumping.

Bad Things Happen to Good People!

When the spine is out of position, it creates abnormal forces not only on the bones, but on the discs between the spinal bones. Stress builds up at the top and bottoms of the vertebrae. This additional stress, causes decreased blood flow to the disc, leading to de-hydration (8).

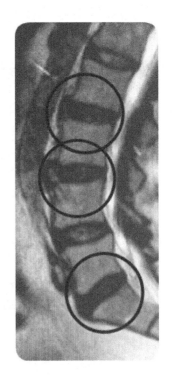

See these black discs (circles).

These are called desiccated discs (de-hydrated or dried-up).

They are precursors to bulges and herniations!

There are 4 bad outcomes that can arise from a dehydrated or dried-up disc. Usually in this order, but not always:

1. Bulging disc

When the disc becomes malnourished it will dry up. This often times causes the walls of the disc to eventually crack (fissure). These cracks allow the jelly material to leak out the back. This is termed a ***bulging disc*** *(see below)*. (9)

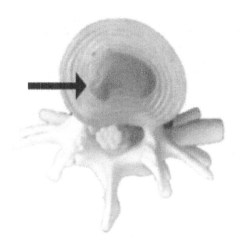

This is what a bulging disc looks like.

The outer ring (annulus) is bulging into the nerve root.

This often times makes the pain go down the leg (sciatic pain).

Look at the MRI below, which shows a bulging disc at L4-L5. This patient had severe pain down the side of their right leg!

This is an MRI of a disc bulge.

You can see the black disc lacks hydration, making it weaker, compared to the white hydrated disc above, which is healthy and strong!

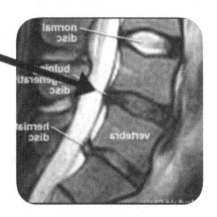

2. Herniated disc

If a portion of the jelly material erupts and comes completely out of the disc, it is referred to as a *herniated disc* (10). Many times, when the disc is herniated, patients go to surgery to have the herniation shaved off. Sometimes the neurosurgeon may be able to shave it without cutting through bone; sometimes not. This disc problem can cause the muscles of the leg to go weak (11), which is a very bad sign!

Herniated disc.

Notice the jelly coming out of the disc right on the nerve!

I had a patient that sneezed while he was on the toilet, of all places, and blew his disc out!

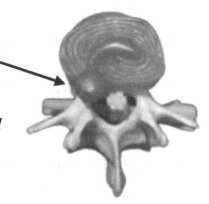

On an MRI it is easy to see the herniation.

This can cause extreme leg pain sometimes without back pain.

It can make the leg muscles go weak.

Some of these go to surgery!

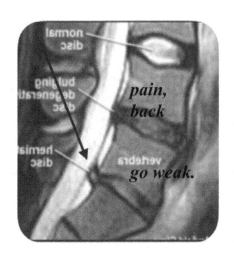

3. Disc collapse

When the disc becomes dried out and weak, it often times starts to collapse (12). This normally happens over a long period of time (roughly 20 years). Many of my patients have both a collapsing and bulging disc.

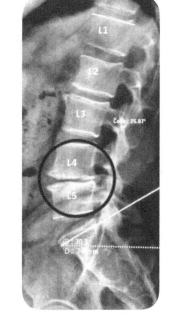

When the disc dries up,

many times, it collapses!

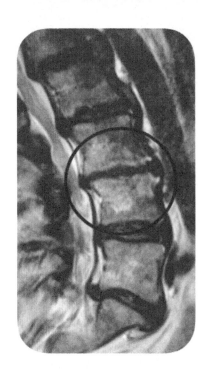

MRI of a collapsed disc with a bulge.

4. Spinal stenosis

When the disc collapses, the spinal bones start to touch each other, causing additional stress on the joints leading to calcium build up. Outcomes of this, include arthritis and bone spurring. Together, this creates a condition known as *stenosis*, which is when the hole where the nerve exits, clogs up with calcium. This results in increased inflammation and pain. Many people who suffer with spinal stenosis will have pain down both legs (13). They often find relief from sitting, because it takes stress off the back part of the spine.

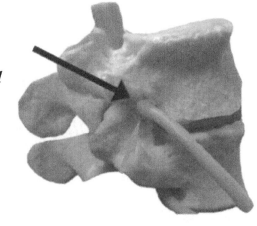

Calcium builds up around the hole where the nerve exits, from too much stress, due to disc loss.

This pinches the nerve.

Don't let that hole get small!!!

Normal spinal nerve openings

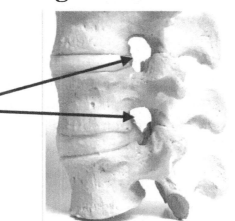

Spinal nerve opening starting to clog up with bone

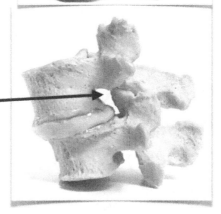

Spinal nerve opening clogged up with bone.

Referred to as stenosis

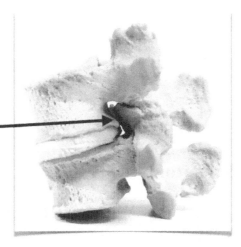

Pain often goes down both legs often relieved by sitting.

In addition, when the disc collapses, the hole where the nerve exits collapses along with it. This results in a pinched nerve, which is the exact reason why people call my office. The most common level the nerve gets pinched is at the very bottom of the spine, L5-S1. This is a weight bearing area, so it is the region that is prone to the greatest stress on it, making it the most likely to be pinched.

Disc bulges, disc herniations and disc collapses all can cause the nerve to get pinched!

When the disc collapses, the hole collapses, pinching the nerve!

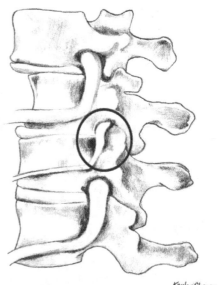

KayleeCheser

The bottom line is this:

YOU DO NOT WANT YOUR DISC TO BE BLACK ON AN MRI!!!

What causes a good disc to dehydrate to begin with?

There are multiple factors, (14) here are Dr. G.'s "Big 6".

1. **Trauma.** Car wrecks, slips and falls, and high impact sports can stress out/injure the disc causing early degeneration.

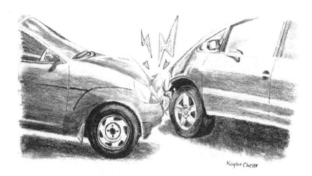

2. **Cumulative trauma**. This comes from excessive bending, lifting, and twisting. People that work on an assembly line or that sit all day, can both jam-up and misalign their spines. This often times will lead to disc dehydration and eventual disc collapse.

3. **Aging**.

When we age the disc becomes less porous, which can cause dehydration and collapse over time.

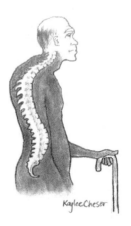

31

4. **Obesity**. Any time you add weight to the spinal joints, the disc will have added pressure which can damage the bottom and tops of the spinal bones. This may cause decreased blood flow to the disc, leading to early degeneration.

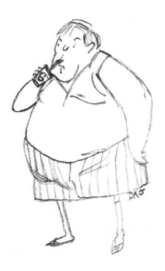

5. Smoking. Nicotine constricts the blood vessels causing poor circulation, leading to dehydration and premature degeneration.

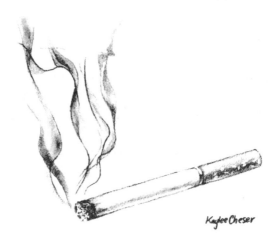

Kaylee Cheser

6. Genetics. A family history of bad backs often times lead to another one in the family tree.

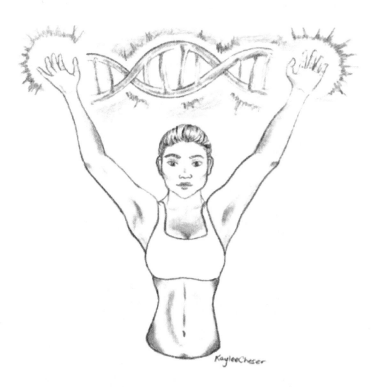

6 Tips for a Healthy Disc!

✓ Keep your spine in great alignment

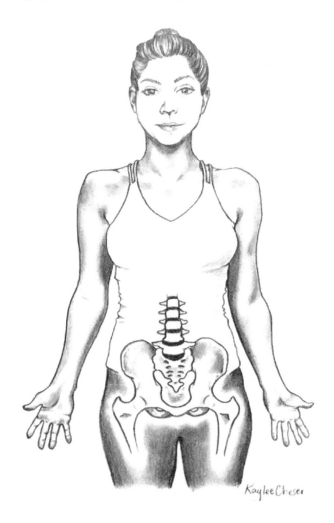

Good alignment of the spine will help remove stress off the vertebrae and discs, helping to keep the good hydration to the inner disc.

These next 7 chapters will teach you how to take care of the spinal alignment and your discs.

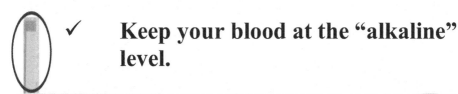

✓ Keep your blood at the "alkaline" level.

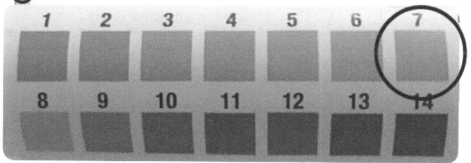

Once you urinate on the pH strip (circled), you immediately compare it to one of the 14 colors. Most people's blood is acidic (1-6).

My wife was all excited because she had an alkaline color #7 (circled).

Our normal body pH is 7.4 which is slightly alkaline. A pH of 7 is neutral. If the body's pH becomes acidic, various alkaline substances including calcium tend to neutralize the excess acid. Therefore, calcium is lost from bones and cartilages, causing the disc to dry up.

These will help raise pH towards 7:

raw foods, especially vegetables

These will lower the pH:

coffee, cigarettes, alcohol, refined sugar, junk food, fast foods, overcooked foods, refined breads, meat

A quick way to check yours is to use pH strips.

You can buy these from Kroger's in the Pharmacy **($32 for 100 strips)**. All you have to do is put a drip of your urine on it and it will change the color of the strip. This will let you know if you are acidic or alkaline.

By the way, I have read numerous articles that say cancer cannot grow in an alkaline environment. (16). My thinking is, if that were 100% truth, then vegetarians (most have alkaline blood) would never get cancer. My belief is that a high pH, is another way among many, to help ward off cancer.

✓ **Exercise**

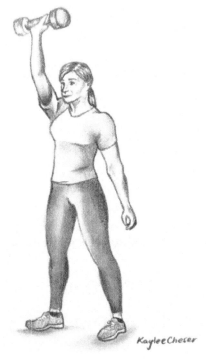

Kaylee Cheser

Regular exercising is very good for the bones, discs and joints. Any form of exercising like walking, yoga, and aerobics is good for the disc. (17)

✓ Weight Reduction

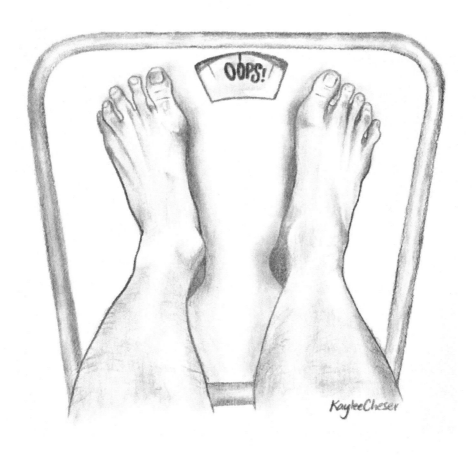

If a person is carrying an excessive amount of weight, over time it will stress out the disc and the joints of the spine. This will lead to early degeneration. Try to keep your weight at an ideal limit for your height. (19)

✓ **Get Plenty of Rest**

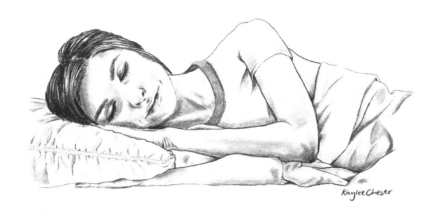

Laying down has the least intradiscal pressure (more on this in Chapter 6). (20) Our discs rehydrate themselves during the night.

The daily dehydration and nightly rehydration of the discs is the reason why most of us are generally about ¼ to ½ inch shorter when we go to bed than when we wake up in the morning! (21)

✓ **Drink plenty of water**. (15)

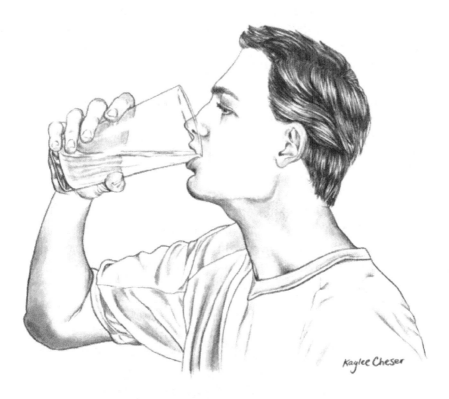

Water is essential for optimum health of the discs.

Best spine of the year goes to Charlie!

As I was about to finish this book, a 91year old gentleman came to my office because he had right hip pain. I was taken aback when I met Charlie because he did not have the presence of a man of nine decades. He was tall and on the slender side. When I patted him on the shoulder when we met, I was shocked because of his muscle tone. As we talked, he told me he hurt his low back three years ago working on his lawn mower, of all things!

When I performed his examination, I was in awe of how far he could bend and twist and just how alert he was. I took two x-rays of his spine. I was amazed when the image of the side of his spine showed up on the computer screen with little to no disc loss or arthritis!

I am often told, but not sold, that everyone's discs are going to wear out with time. Charlie is just one of the cases that prove that there are exceptions to this way of thinking. Some of this may be genetic, but I would make a stronger case that it is environmental. I believe Charlie has been smart his whole life about taking care of his frame and now it is paying huge dividends because he is enjoying his great health, everyday!

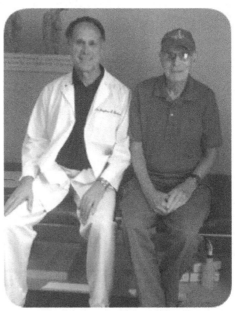

Me and Charlie!

Best spine of the year award!

A side view of 91-year old, Charlie!

Look at how thick his discs are! There is hardly any wear and tear!

This is one of the reasons he can work out in the garden all day!

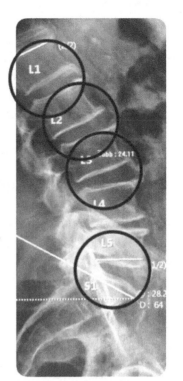

A side view of another 91-year old.

The bottom 3 discs are completely collapsed. The other 2 are collapsing.

She is using a cane and can barely get around.

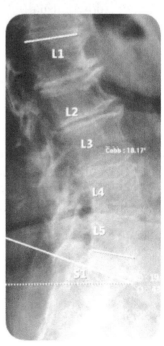

Take Home Message

✓ The disc's primary purpose is to give shock absorption to the spine, provide flexibility to the vertebral column, and to provide space for the outgoing nerve.

✓ A healthy disc is fully hydrated (70-80% water). Hydrated discs as a rule are thick, and the jelly material is usually in the middle. On an MRI, the healthy discs are white.

✓ When the spine is out of alignment, abnormal stresses can build up on the bottoms and tops (end plates) of the vertebra. This can cause a decrease in blood flow to the disc. As a result, the disc breaks down (cracks) and the jelly material starts to <u>bulge</u> out the back of the disc. Often times, this can put pressure on the nerve.

✓ A <u>herniated</u> disc occurs when the wall of the disc breaks down, usually from a dried out (desiccated) disc, and leaks out the back. This condition, many times, will cause extreme pain down the leg to the foot. Surgeons often times, will have to remove the disc material.

✓ A collapsed disc occurs when there is period of time, usually 20+ years, of continued abnormal stress on the disc. I often see this condition from an old car accident. When the disc collapses, the space collapses where the nerve exits. This can cause not only back pain, but leg pain on one or both sides. On MRI they are usually black.

✓ A few ways to keep the disc healthy are: good alignment, alkaline pH, exercise, weight reduction, rest, and hydration.

STEP 1

H2O-Not a Cup of Jo

"Water is the only drink for a wise man."
-Henry David Thoreau

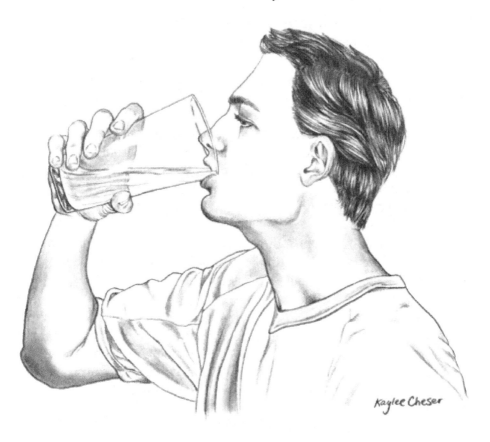

Kaylee Cheser

Nightmare at the Outback Steakhouse!

Tony, a sixty-year-old male, entered my clinic as his back pain had flared up again. This was the exact same pain he was battling with two years ago. Before we started the examination, he asked me if he could tell me a story about what had happened to him a few months ago.

He said he, his wife, and another couple were dining at Outback Steakhouse in Clarksville, Indiana. After they got their meal, he started getting dizzy and getting pains in his chest. He said that he felt like his face was about ready to drop right on his 12-ounce ribeye.

He muttered to his wife to call 9-1-1. Shortly afterwards, EMS was at their table in the Outback trying to revive him. They transported him on a gurney to the ambulance where they tested him only to find out he was dehydrated. They inserted an IV into his vein to get him rehydrated.

The paramedic asked him what he drank that day and he said coffee in the morning, and two liters of cola in the afternoon. They asked him if he had any water of which he said, he had not. He went on to explain his typical liquid diet was primarily coffee in the morning and a couple liters of cola a day, with little to no water!

He explained to Tony that the coffee and cola had dehydrated him to the point his body was starting to shut down. In addition, he told him to replace his coffee and cola habit with water!

Since the day after his close call, by and large his only liquids have been water! Within thirty days, he said that he could bend further and felt more flexible than he had in years! He went on to tell me that ten years earlier he could out drive all his friends on the golf course, but the last 5 or so years his friends were out driving him. However, this last month he was back to hitting the ball further than his friends again. An extra 30 yards was added to his drive from rehydrating his body!

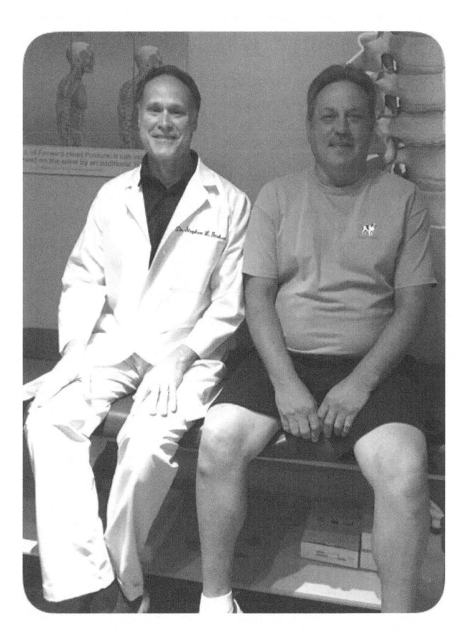

Tony got off his cola habit and is only taking in water!

He said he is driving the golf ball 30 yards further since he changed his habit!

Why are soft drinks so bad?

It is not just that soft drinks cause diabetes, obesity, and the teeth to rot, but people will only ingest so many liquids a day and it takes away from proper hydrating opportunities. In addition, anything with caffeine, which soft drinks have, are a diuretic if ingested in excess.

A rule of thumb is more than a couple soft drinks a day and more than 500mg of coffee (approximately 4 cups) may cause you to lose sodium which will contribute to dehydration.

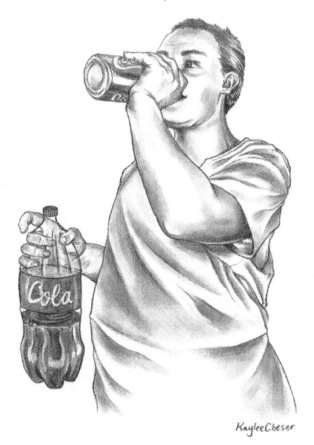

KayleeCheser

Soft drinks are contributors to disc dehydration!

Why do we need to hydrate in the first place?

The reason we need to take hydration seriously is because our bodies are made up of 65% water.

- brain and heart - 73%
- lungs - 83%
- skin - 64%
- muscles and kidneys - 79%
- **discs- 80%**
- bones are 31% (1)

Ways we get hydrated

The typical person gets 80% of their hydration from liquids and 20% from food. Our bodies use this water for digestion, blood, tears, mucous, saliva, lubrication, synovial fluids for joints, and disc hydration. The disc gets hydrated two ways: imbibition and sleep.

Imbibition: Water pumped in disc

The intervertebral disc requires plenty of water and nutrients to stay healthy and perform at its best, just like the rest of our body. However, the problem is, that as early as five years of age, the spinal discs lose the nutritional supply coming from blood. (1) Therefore, at an early age, the spine is only able to receive water and nutrients through osmosis, a process called ***imbibition.*** Imbibition occurs when there is normal motion between each vertebra. This movement acts as a pump, moving water in and out of each disc.

Imbibition:

Water pumped in disc for rehydration

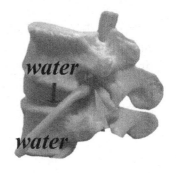

water

water

So, when there is adequate water in the body and normal spine movement, the result is good rehydration of the disc.

Rehydration while we sleep

During the course of the day, all the compressive forces from sitting or standing, cause the disc to lose water and shrink. When we get out of gravity (sleeping) the disc rehydrates, through osmosis, some or all of the lost fluid that was lost that day. The regained fluid, provides sometimes, up to a half inch more of height upon waking.

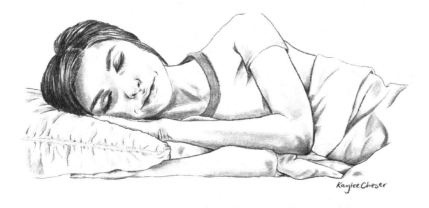

Kaylee Cheser

This same force is at work when astronauts travel to outer space. According to NASA research, astronauts gain up to two inches in height once they are freed from the gravitational pressure of earth. Because we don't live on the moon, the force of the earth's gravity compresses our spines throughout the day, draining that extra fluid and shrinking height that extra half-inch. (2)

How do we get dehydrated?

We get dehydrated when our water losses are higher than our water intake. Here is a list of some quick ways to lose water: not drinking enough, vigorous exercise, vomiting, diarrhea, excessive sweating, diuretics (excessive caffeine drinks), alcohol, and medications.

Symptoms that you may be dehydrated include: thirst, dry mouth, nausea, fatigue, lightheadedness, darkened and decreased urine, irritability, difficulty concentrating, and headaches.

Long-term effects from chronic dehydration are the following:

- Digestive disturbances such as heartburn and constipation
- Urinary tract infections
- Autoimmune disease such as chronic fatigue syndrome and multiple sclerosis
- Premature aging
- High cholesterol
- Weight gain
- **Degenerative disc disease**

How does this affect my back?

When you are not hydrated properly, it forces your body to make some pretty tough decisions, such as pulling moisture from "low priority" areas to protect vital functions. ABC's News chief health and medical editor, Dr. Richard Besser explained to Good Morning America, "If you get dehydrated, your body is going to pull water from other tissues, such as your skin, to maintain the concentration in your blood." Besser shared that when this happens, it leaves your skin drier and less elastic.

Other tissues of low priority are the tendons and ligaments. One such ligament is the intervertebral disc. So, just like the skin, when there is low hydration, the body will rob Peter (disc) to pay Paul (blood). What this means for the back is, the discs may dry out. If there is already a deficiency present, then there will be no excess water to rehydrate the discs of the spine. This, more than likely, will lead to disc bulges, herniations and collapse!

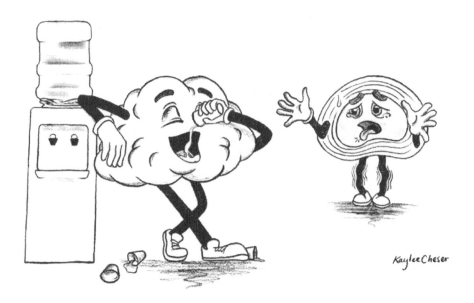

The brain, cardiovascular system, and lungs get first dibs with the water you ingest, while the ligaments and discs are in the back of the line!

Let's look at Tony's intervertebral discs.

See how his bottom two discs are dehydrated and collapsed.

Did all his lack of hydration and all the soda for so many years cause this?

Probably not all, but maybe some of it.

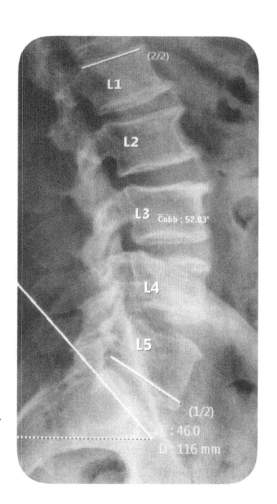

Exactly how much water should we ingest to keep our body and discs properly hydrated?

There is a rule of thumb that I learned in chiropractic school. The formula is to take your body weight and divide it by two. That number, is the number of ounces of water you should drink per day!

$$\frac{Body\ Weight}{2} = ounces\ of\ hydration\ per\ day$$

So, if Jane weighs 150 pounds, she should drink 75 ounces of water. For me, since I weigh 180 pounds, I should be drinking 90 ounces of water.

What Type of Water is Best!

I have been a practicing chiropractor for over twenty-five years. During this time, I have heard all the hype there is about the different types of water. It can be very easy to get confused about which type of water is the best, from the dangerous chemicals in tap water to the environmental concerns of bottled water.

If you want to cut through all the clutter, I would highly recommend reading about this on Dr. Joseph Mercola's website (Mercola.com). Dr. Mercola is a doctor of Osteopathy and New York Times best-selling author. He has great researched articles about this very topic. I would suggest you read his work because I know him to be very knowledgeable in this confusing area of healthy living.

I have briefly outlined on the following page what he talks about in his research.

Tap water is contaminated with the following chemicals:

1. **"Arsenic**: This poisonous element is a powerful carcinogenic, which has been linked to an increased risk of the development of several types of cancer. (4)

2. **Aluminum**: Aluminum has been linked to:

- Hyperactivity
- Learning disabilities in children
- Gastrointestinal disease
- Skin problems
- Parkinson's disease
- Liver disease (4)

3. **Fluoride**: This toxin weakens your immune system and accelerates aging due to cellular damage. (4)

4. **Prescription and OTC drugs (coming from landfills and toilets):** Pregnant women should be especially wary. The toxic substances you take into your body from tap water may have a negative effect on the development of your unborn child. (4)

5. **Disinfection Byproducts (DBPs):** Disinfection byproducts are the result of disinfecting water with chlorine. In addition to a powerful carcinogenic, DPBs have also been linked to liver, kidney and nervous system problems." (4)

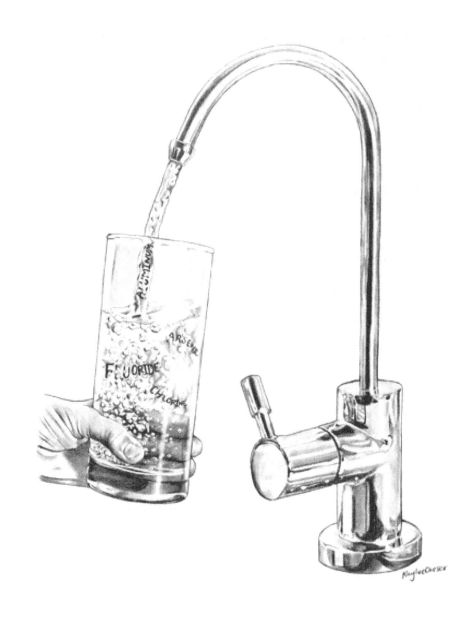

Arsenic, Aluminum, Fluoride, Chlorine and Aluminum are all found in our tap water!

Bottled Water

40 percent of bottled water is TAP WATER!

"40 percent of bottled water is just bottled tap water, which may or may not have received additional filtration. Remember the arsenic and DPBs you were trying to avoid from tap water? Well, an independent test done by the Environmental Working Group found these and 36 other harmful pollutants hidden in bottled water." (4)

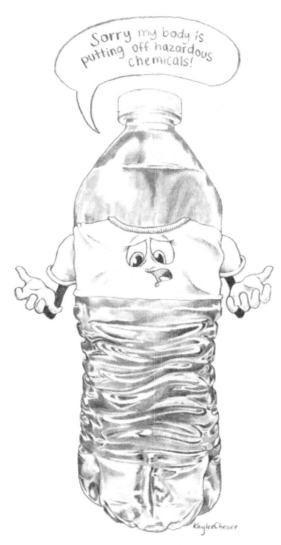

"Also, drinking from plastic bottles is not a good idea. Plastic bottles contain a chemical called bisphenol A or BPA, which is a synthetic hormone disruptor that has been linked to serious health problems such as:

- Learning and behavioral problems
- Altered immune system function
- Prostate and breast cancer
- Risk of obesity
- Early puberty in both genders

Aside from the health risks, the devastating impact bottled water has had on our ecosystem is staggering!" (4)

Filtered Tap Water

The most economical and environmentally sound choice you and your family can make is to purchase a water filter system for your home. Below are three economical ones.

Reverse Osmosis Filter:

This filter removes chlorine, inorganic, organic contaminants in your water, and about 80 percent of the fluoride and most DPBs.

Ion Exchange Filter

Typically, about 95% of known water contaminants are dissolved inorganics, such as calcium. So, processes that remove ions can potentially remove up to about 95% of all the contaminants.

Granular Carbon and Carbon Block Filters

These are the most common types of counter top and under counter water filters. Granular activated carbon is recognized by the EPA as the best available technology for the removal of organic chemicals like herbicides, pesticides and industrial chemicals.

Health Benefits of Drinking Filtered Water

Here are some of the benefits when you switch from tap or bottled water to filtered water:

- a healthier body-weight
- better food digestion and absorption of nutrients
- healthier, glowing skin
- decreased muscle and joint inflammation
- better circulation
- improved detoxification (4)

I Bought a "Berkey"

I have had at least four filtration systems in the last 25 years, but I like the "Berkey Water System" the best! In fact, not only do I have one at home ("Baby Berkey"), but I also purchased one to use at work ("Big Berkey"). I feel that at least I am being responsible to my staff, my patients and myself, by filtering out 99% of the contaminates.

These units are about $250 but will filter 1000 gallons before you need to change the filter. Smart money says for that many gallons of chemical free water, it is nothing short of a bargain!

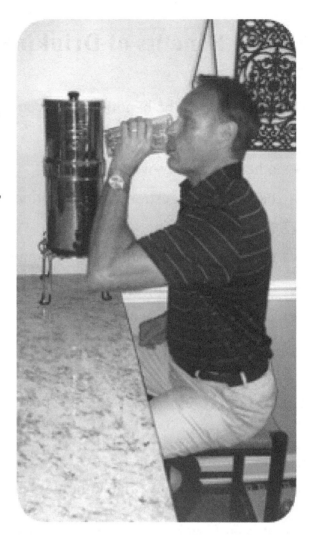

Me, drinking my first 20 ounces of filtered water in the morning, right out of my Berkey Water System!

Great way to start my day!

Each morning I wake up, I drink 20 ounces of filtrated water and am well on my way to getting hydrated. When I get to work, I drink from my Big Berkey all morning and pretty much without fail, I have ingested most of my 90 ounces of great purified water by noon. On my most active days, I like to add another 16 ounces.

Take Home Message

✓ <u>Our disc is last in line to get a drink.</u> This means if we really want a healthy back we have to be intentional on our daily hydration. We cannot have a large consumption of coffee and other caffeinated beverages and expect to not end up with a potential disc problem.

✓ <u>Consume half of your body weight in ounces</u> to ensure that you are achieving the proper daily hydration. In addition, if you are active you will need to go above and beyond that because you are sweating and using more hydration than a non-active person.

✓ <u>Get a water filtration system.</u> This will ensure that you are not getting contaminates in your water that can make you get sick or age prematurely. You can buy a good system that removes 95% of the contaminates for around $200-250. Remember any filtration system is better than tap or bottled water!

STEP 2

It's the Core

If one part suffers, every part suffers with it;
if one part is honored, every part rejoices with it.

-1Corinthians 12:26

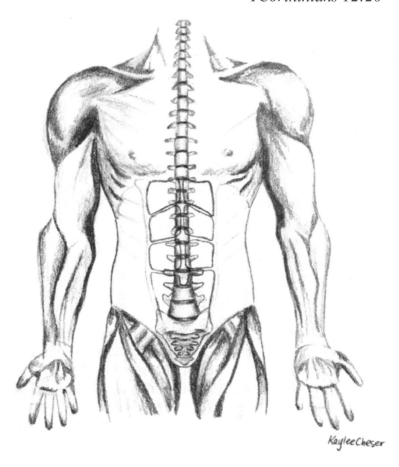

KayleeCheser

Four Chin-Ups...You Can't Be Serious!

In 1973, I was a young freshman at Trinity High school. For the first two weeks in gym class, 30 guys competed against each other in the Presidential Physical Fitness Test. From what I can recall, there were four or five tests including sit ups, softball throw, 50-yard dash, and chin ups. It was fun seeing how I stacked up against the other 14-year-olds, mostly coming from surrounding Catholic grade schools around Louisville. I especially remember the chin up competition, because we were all in a big room and one by one, everyone had a chance to show their stuff on the chin up bar in front of the entire class.

Me as a freshman, looking way too serious!

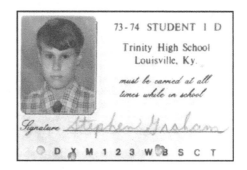

There were a handful in our class that could not do one chin up. I was feeling for them as they were being made fun of, as 14-year-olds can do. I only managed a measly four, which was not much better. I remember Ray Vanover popped up 16 times! It looked as if it was almost effortless, and pretty much made me sick. As he got to 10 with plenty of steam left, I began thinking how pitiful I was, but it did motivate me to start doing these in my basement!

As I look back on these events, each one was a test of the strength of my core muscles. The sit ups focused on the muscles in my stomach; the softball throw worked my obliques; the 50-yard dash taxed my obliques and gluteus maximus; and the chin ups targeted primarily my biceps, but while I was hanging in the air, the muscles that create the six pack, were working to keep my body in a straight line.

I am not suggesting for you to try your hand at the Presidential Fitness Test today or any other day, but you get the idea that to do well in athletics, you must have a strong core.

And to have a good strong back you must have a fit core, as well. Since a weak torso is such a common finding in my examinations, I am devoting a whole chapter just to the CORE!

What in the heck is the core?

Because we walk on two legs rather than four, our back right off the bat, becomes one of the weak links of our human anatomy. Our spine needs constant help from its supporting muscles to minimize the load on the spine. With no muscle support (tested on dead bodies) the back can only bear loads up to 5 pounds without collapsing. (1) With well-developed torso muscles or core, the spine can take loads up to 2000 pounds (one ton). That's a 400-fold increase! (1)

The core consists of the muscles in the front and back of the lower spine, as well as those wrapping around the sides. Together, these help not only to protect and support the spine, but to keep it in good alignment.

Let's take a look at the:

core muscles-front and side: rectus abdominis and oblique muscles (see illustration on next page) (2),

and

core muscles-back: erector spinae, quadratus lumborum, and gluteus maximus muscles (see illustration on next page) (2):

Front and side "Core"

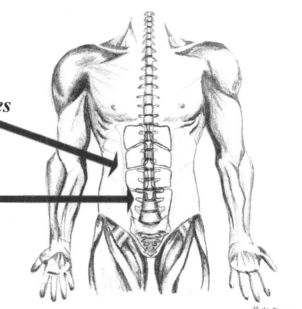

- *Oblique Muscles*

- *Rectus Abdominis Muscle, also known as the "six pack"*

Back "Core"

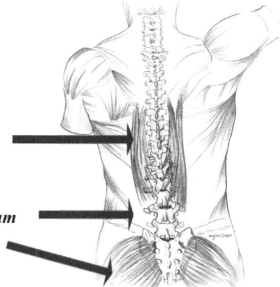

- *Erector Spinae*

- *Quadratus Lumborum*
- *Gluteus Maximus*

As I mentioned in the previous chapter, the frontal view of the spine should appear straight, but while looking at the spine from the side, it should be arch shaped, like the x-ray below.

Better Core = Better Alignment.

Correct and strongest <u>angulation</u> is 45 degrees.

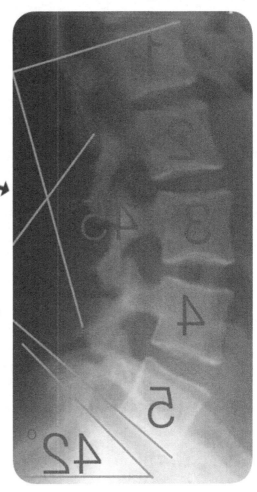

A strong core is more likely to keep the spine in this alignment!

My experience tells me, if you have a good core, accompanied with a correctly aligned spine, you will exponentially reduce your risk of ever developing back pain.

Bad Core = Bad Alignment

Many patients have asked me how they would know if they have a weak core. Everyone is unique, but these are four signs of a weak core (4):

1. Back pain. If the muscles surrounding your spine are weak, the vertebrae and discs of your spine will not be properly supported. This will probably cause you to experience back pain at some point.

2. Poor posture. The muscles of your abdomen and lower back combine to hold your spine and pelvis in place. If these muscles are weak, your body may be unstable causing you difficulty to sit or stand straight for more than a short period without back pain.

3. Bad balance. Your core muscles stabilize your entire body, so a weak core will affect your ability to balance. To test this, stand on one leg for 10 seconds; if it is too difficult to hold this, you probably have an underdeveloped core.

4. Overweight. If you are 25 pounds or more overweight, you may have a weakened core.

A Weak Core Contributes to IT Specialist's Back Pain!

Case Study

Recently, a 41-year-old man consulted me about a pain in his lower back. He explained that his pains were in his central lower back and it radiated down the back of his right leg all the way to his ankle. Occasionally, he experienced numbness in his foot.

As I began to do the eye ball test across the table, it became very evident that he had let things go physically in his life. Exercise, I am sure, was not even close to being on his radar. He was probably thirty pounds overweight, with very little tone in his body. He was an IT specialist by trade, so he sat for 6-8 hours every day. Three or four times a week he told me he ate lunch at his desk and consumed 4-6 Ibuprofen daily. This regimen has been consistent for the last two or so years.

His case was a great example of how low back pain is directly related to a weakened core. His abdominal muscles had not been activated probably since college and his glute muscles were flaccid. When I looked at his x-ray, his spine sagged (see below), because his core muscles were not getting the job done.

You can see below that this sagging caused a sharp angle in the small of his back, or in doctors speak, at L5-S1. This led to abnormal forces being exerted on his lower spine, ultimately causing a desiccated, bulging disc at L5-S1. This was confirmed by the MRI he brought in (see next page-circled area).

60.88 degrees

Way too much angulation!

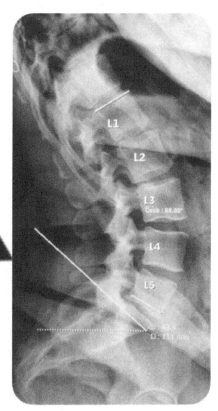

His MRI shows a dried-up bulging disc

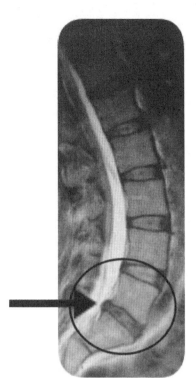

This man fell into this all too common category: "All I do is work, eat, watch TV, and sleep", a group that is on an upward trend because of computers, video games and Netflix. Interestingly, this category as a whole, is usually surprised that their back hurts. Often times these same people tell me that they have not done anything. And they are right. They have not done anything, for their core, that is!

Gave him a core exercise, which he actually did!

After discussing his correction schedule of spinal adjustments, I went over his new exercise program. The way I up the odds in getting a patient to be compliant, is to give him or her one thing to do, rather than ten things. So, I gave him one core exercise to do at home. After two weeks of realigning his spine and him working doing his one core exercise, his lower back and leg pain began to subdue.

Core Exercises

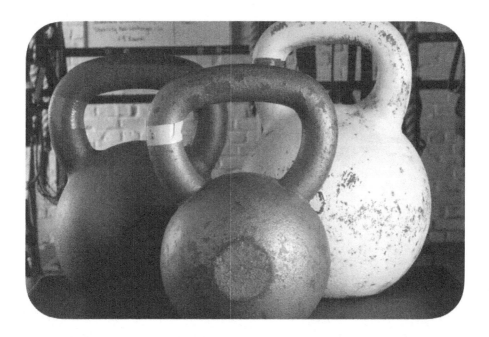

"Dr. G, are there 3 or 4 simple things I can do that only take 10 minutes, because my time is so limited with work and activities, that I barely have time to get on Facebook for two hours every day?"

The answer to that is yes. I have <u>four exercises</u> that are easy and in time will develop your core (5).

1. ***Planks.*** Lay down on the floor and prop yourself up with your elbows keeping your body in a straight line. **Hold this for 30 seconds**. If you can only do it for 5 seconds, great. Just do that for now and increase your time, as your core gets stronger.

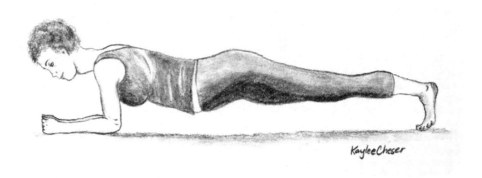

KayleeCheser

2. ***Abdominal crunches.*** Lay on your back with your knees bent. Gently put your hands on the side of your head and slowly lift up your head, neck, and upper back off the floor focusing on using your core to raise you. Inhale on the way up and exhale on the way down. **Do 3 sets of 10 with a minute break between sets.**

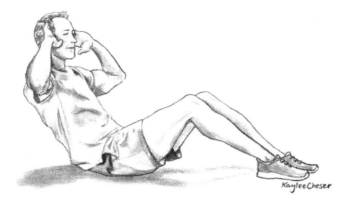

KayleeCheser

3. **_Push-ups._** I would highly recommend doing these with your knees on the floor to begin with or standing and pushing off from a counter top. You can always build up to "big boy" push-ups, but let's keep the main thing, the main thing, by not getting hurt when you are trying to get healthy!

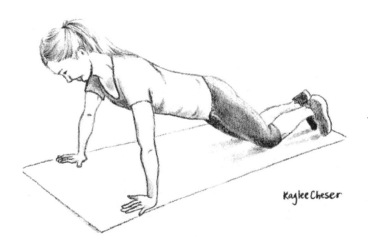

Do 3 sets of 10 with a minute break between sets.

4. *Lunges for your glutes.* One leg is positioned forward with knee bent and foot flat on the ground, while the other leg is positioned behind. **Do 10 lunges one time**. I really like this one!

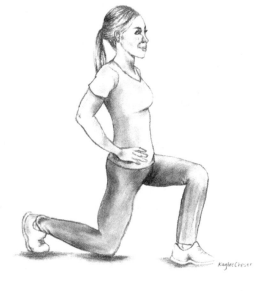

Dr. G. likes this one!

71

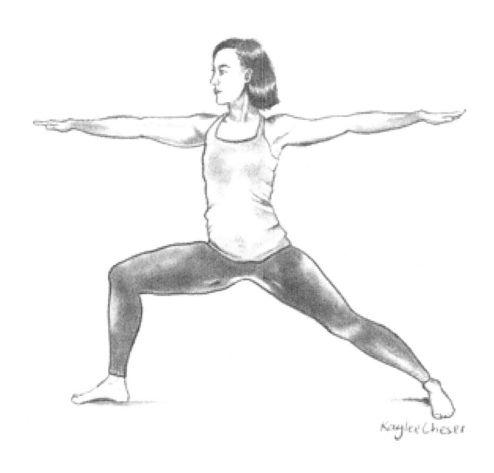

Kaylee Cheser

Bonus exercise: Warrior yoga pose.

The warrior pose is a great exercise that will tax your core.

"Dr. G, those exercises look like fun and all, but I am 80 years old! What can I do, because I sure as heck can't do those?"

Glad you asked, here is my "Easy 3"!

By the way, you can be younger than 80 and start with these.

#1. *Standing one arm dumbbell exercises.* The point of these is the side that does not have weight on it will contract to keep the body in alignment. I personally like the standing one arm curl and the standing press (below). **Do ten of each on both sides.**

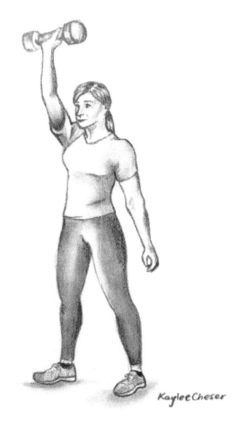

Kaylee Cheser

#2. Air squats.

Hold onto
something firm
and squat
bending your
knees about half
way. **Do 1 set of
5-10.**

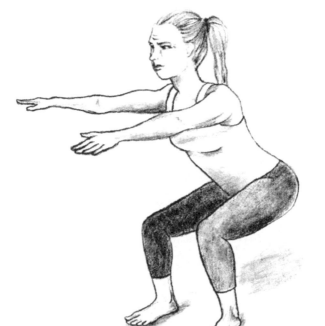

#3. Push-ups off a wall

Do 10 of these one time,
keeping your body in straight
alignment.

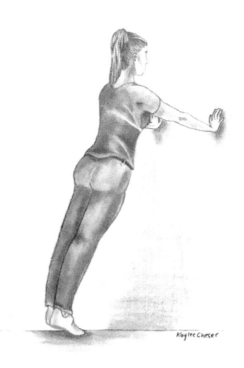

Good Housekeeping

Correct technique is a must during exercise as it will maximize your benefit and lower your risk of injury. This is in contrast to poor exercise form, which increases the possibility of injury and diminishes results. I have had many patients come from the gym who reported that they had injured their back from poor technique (dead lifts keep me in business!).

The benefits to the spine from a well-built core include (6):

1. **Better alignment**
2. **Increased back strength**
3. **Greater endurance**
4. **Wider range of flexibility**
5. **More efficient function**
6. **Improved mobility**

These will offset the risk of back pain by an off the charts percentage!

The idea I have for most people, is not to achieve six pack abs, but is just to wake your core up and slap it into better shape. If you are a patient in my office, make sure you check with me first before doing any core exercises. Likewise, if you are not a patient, check with someone who is a professional. Again, remember to keep the main focus on not getting hurt!

Now I am talking to the 10 percenters!

I have done kettlebells in the past and for a guy in his 50's, I am not sure that I want to tackle these now. I am pretty happy with the easier regime I do now. One important concept I have learned over my years is, <u>don't mess with happy</u>!

But, if you want to take on a harder challenge for your core...

...kettlebells (7) are an extremely effective type of exercise to increase functional strength, endurance, and flexibility in the entire body, but especially to the core muscles. During kettlebell training, the core muscles will stabilize the body, so you can develop the smaller supporting muscles.

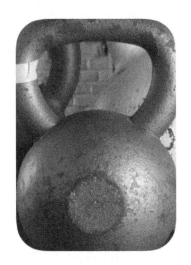

25 lb. kettle bell

Usually with the higher reward exercises, there comes a higher risk. So, while kettlebells are great for the core they do pose a larger threat for injury.

TIP from Dr. G: I really like the benefits of deadlifts, but the risk of a disc injury is very high compared to most other exercises.

A great substitute for these are called suitcase deadlifts (below) which gives most of the same benefits of a deadlift, with much less risk!

Suitcase deadlifts

Much, much less risky than standard deadlifts.

My wife reluctantly agreed to be photographed for this!

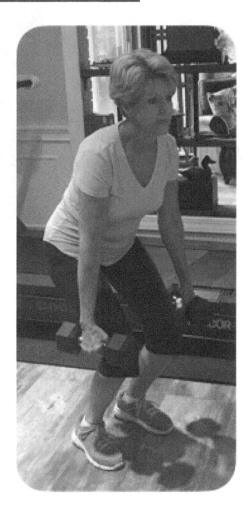

New APP for the person on the go!

Many years ago, I would have to go the health and fitness racks at the local Barnes and Noble to find some new exercises, but in 2018 all you have to do is go to the APP search and find whatever your heart desires. Last year I was introduced to "Bodyweight Training".

Great APP!

Everyone should have this on their phone!

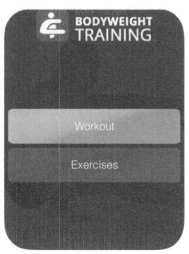

This is an APP, not a book, and all the exercises involve moving the weight of your body. I especially like this, because you don't need to have a gym membership. This APP is designed for busy people in mind, who may only have 5 minutes to work out. I challenge you to try it out!

So good luck and don't forget....

...a better core = a better spine!

Take Home Message

✓ There are front, side and back core muscles that help to support your spine.

The front and side core muscles include: the *abs and the obliques*. The core muscles of the back include: the *erector spinae, latissimus dorsi and the gluteus maximus*.

✓ A strong core keeps the spine from sagging in the lower back. This sag puts excessive stress on the low back joints which can lead to disc loss, arthritis and pain.

✓ There are 4 signs that your core may be weak. These are: back pain, poor posture, bad balance, carrying extra weight.

✓ These exercises improve the core: *planks, push-ups, sit-ups (with knees bent), walking, one armed dumbbell exercises*. For more advanced core training, try out *kettle bells*.

Step 3

Build Your Arch
Before it Rains

*And the rain fell, and the floods came, and the winds blew
and beat on that house, but it did not fall,
because it had been founded on the rock.*
-Matthew 7:25

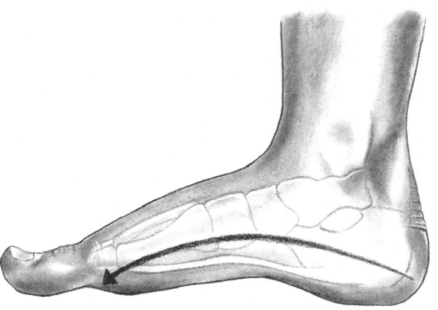

Kaylee Chiser

It's about the Keystone!

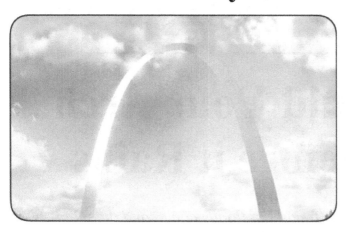

As I was driving across I-64 destined for St. Louis to attend Logan College of Chiropractic, there was a large cluster of trees on my left at mile marker nine. As I made my way past the towering trees, suddenly, in all its majesty, I could see the shiny St. Louis Arch! It stood tall, monumental, and magnificent, all 630 feet of it! And this was at nine miles outside of the city!

It seemed as though every time my friends came to visit, they wanted to visit the arch. As many times that I have taken the tour, I believe I could give it myself. The one part of the tour that I remembered most, was the video showing the construction process. The crescendo of the documentary was when they filmed the very last block being inserted, the keystone. It was the single block that anchored the entire arch. As Leonardo da Vinci brilliantly stated, "the keystone brings together two weaknesses to make a strength"!

From an engineering standpoint, an arch is advantageous because it transfers and balances the load instead of focusing it on one spot. That is why the arch is the strongest structure known to mankind.

In addition to its strength, they present stability and beauty. Arches are often designed for doorways, buildings, bridges, and even add a magical passageway for entrances such as Yellowstone National Park; Arc de Triomphe; and even Bellarmine University, my alma mater!

Have you ever wondered how, our foot, such a small part of the body, can handle the weight of our entire frame?

It is because our feet are designed with arches. The arch of the foot is the greatest weight bearing design ever created. Naturally this arch has a keystone as well, the Talus bone.

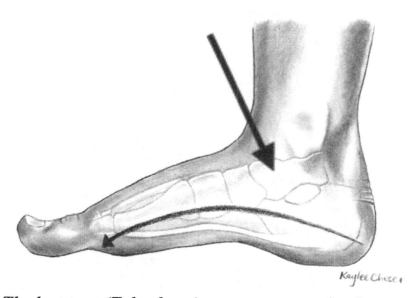

The keystone (Talus bone) supports our entire frame.

You may question the importance and wonder why I am talking about feet, when this book is about the back. Here is why: the feet are the foundation of our whole body, when the arches are in good alignment, then the alignment of the lumbar spine (lower back) is usually healthier.

3 Arches, not 1!

There are three arches in the foot. The main arch that most people think of is the inside arch or medial arch. However, there are two more arches. The second arch is the outside arch or lateral arch. Finally, there is the transverse arch which is under the top third of the foot. These three arches join together to create the "Plantar Vault" in our foot.

The arches job is to dissipate all the forces from running and walking, and when the foot has a good vault it will absorb these impacts all day long!

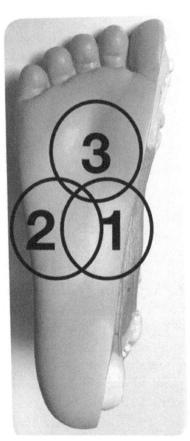

A normal foot has 3 arches, not 1.

1 = Medial arch

2 = Lateral arch

3 = Transverse arch

Together they create the "Plantar Vault".

How do you know if your feet have good arches?

There are a few easy ways to do this. The simplest way is to just get your feet wet, step out on the sidewalk and look at the imprint.

Normal footprints have a gap where the arches are raised from the ground, in contrast to collapsed arches, which will show most of the bottom of the foot. Here is an example of a good arch:

This person has great arches.

Notice how only about half the foot is in contact with the ground.

This is an indicator that a person's back pain is not influenced by a fallen arch.

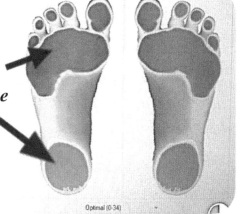

The above picture is a laser image of the feet. This technology was developed by FootLevelers **(see page 83).** It is easy to see that a high, healthy arch has only about half of the foot in contact with the surface. This is a clear sign that the forces of the step are being 100% absorbed by the Plantar Vault. In addition, good arches help the legs to stay in good alignment which help to balance the pelvis.

Since the spine rests on the pelvis, good arches will also help to keep the spine straighter, decreasing the chances of back pain. **See diagram on next page:**

Straight Man

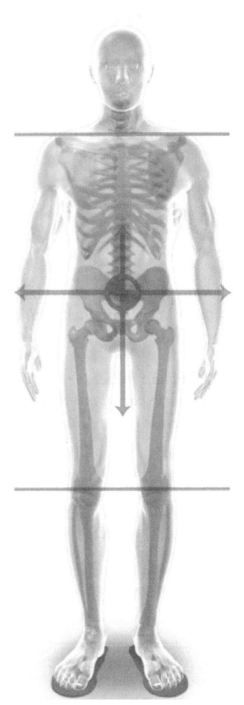

See how the legs are evenly aligned because the arches are not fallen.

Due to the legs proper alignment, the pelvis is level and balanced.

The leveled pelvis helps to keep the spine straight, reducing the chance of back pain!

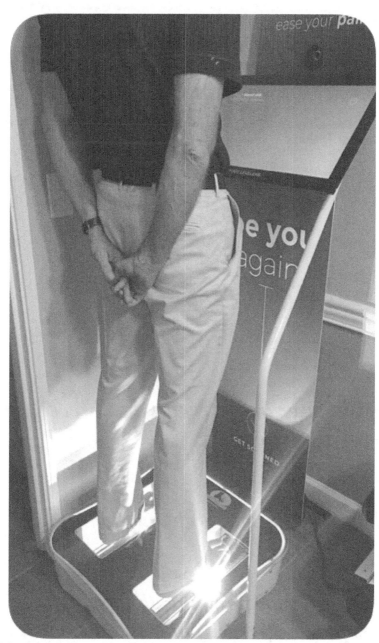

This laser image is accurate up to 1 micron.

The image will tell if each step taken, is or is not, transferring impact up the kinetic chain to the knees, hips and spine.

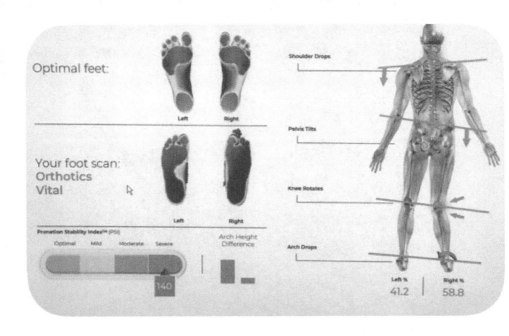

This is a laser image report that I receive on each of my patients.

It shows the normal arch and their arch.

The report also shows the abnormal stress that is put on specific joints in the body if the arches are collapsing, such as the knee, hip and spine.

Bad Arches

When the arches in the foot collapse the forces are not totally absorbed by the Plantar Vault. **The forces that are not dissipated by the 3 arches, are transferred up the kinetic chain to the knee, hip and the low back!**

This may result in additional stress on the vertebral disc, leading to degeneration and back problems. (1) **See next page.**

What causes the arch to collapse?

Exercise (running, jumping, dancing), sports (basketball, volley- ball, etc.), jobs that require excessive time spent on the feet, or wearing poorly supportive shoes can cause damage to the tendons in the foot. (2)

A fallen arch is more commonly found in women and people over 40 years of age. (3)

Additional risk factors include, obesity, diabetes, rheumatoid arthritis, broken or dislocated foot bones.

Genetics may also play a role **(see page 91).**

Crooked Man

A fallen arch can cause the leg, pelvis and lumbar spine to move out of alignment.

This often times leads to back pain.

If the doctor does not look for a collapsing arch, the cause may go undetected.

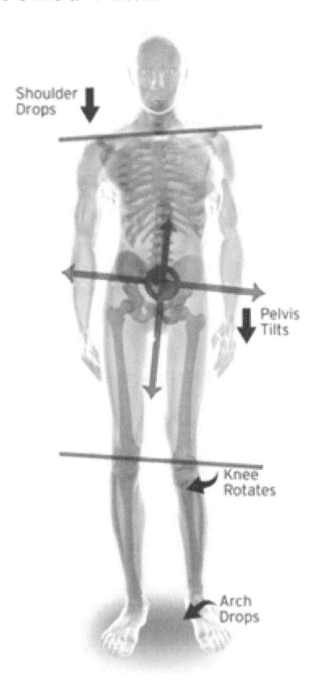

Shoulder Drops

Pelvis Tilts

Knee Rotates

Arch Drops

Genetics can play a role! Look at this family.

Mom

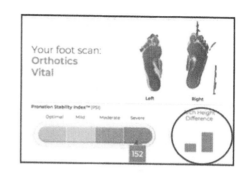

Daughter #1

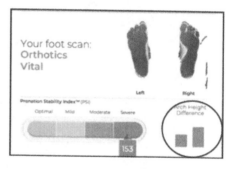

Daughter #2

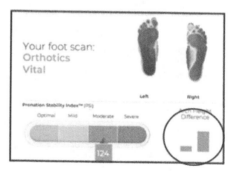

Each family member has a severely collapsed left arch.

All three came to my office for back pain!

Warning signs that you may have a fallen arch.

1. Pain in the bottom of the foot (5)
2. Knee rotation (5)
3. Bowed Achilles tendon (5)
4. Uneven shoe wear (5)

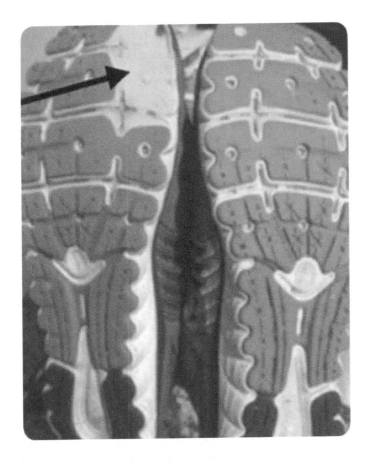

Uneven wear on the soles.

It is common for a person with a collapsed arch to have knee pain on the same side.

What does someone do with an arch that goes bad?

I think the most prudent thing to do is to **wear a good pair of orthotics in your shoes to help raise the arch.** This will:

1. sequentially help to realign the legs, hips, and spine, which will help to…

2. …remove forces transferring to the knees and spine from the unabsorbed forces from a pronated foot.

All orthotics are not made equal

Custom Orthotics

Years ago, Denny Crum, University of Louisville's Hall of Fame former basketball coach, used to be the pitchman for Super Feet. Super Feet are a hard orthotic that commercials advertised as the answer to many ailments, including back pain. Many of my patients, including myself, were disillusioned by the discomfort the hard plastic afforded. Because of this, they quit wearing them.

In the early 2000's, I went to a Foot Levelers seminar. I was highly impressed with the scientific research behind their orthotics and was equally impressed with the technology that went in to measuring the arch of the foot. I prescribe Foot Levelers to many of my patients. Some of them reported feeling the stress immediately come off their back. The majority of patients wearing these orthotics, stated that their spinal adjustments held longer.

Low back pain reduced 34.5% simply by wearing FootLevelers, a 3-Arched orthotic.

In 2017, a randomized control trial was published in the *Archives of Physical Medicine* that proved that Foot Levelers custom-made orthotics reduced low back pain by 34.5%

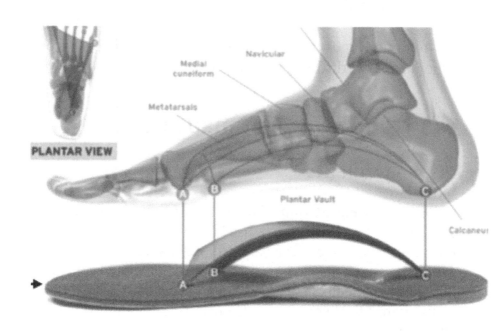

Foot Levelers Custom Orthotic

Website: Footlevelers.com

Is Your Spine Resting on a Solid Foundation?

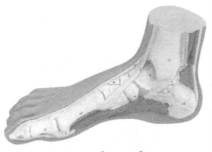

normal arch

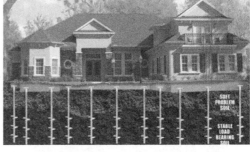

Firm Foundation

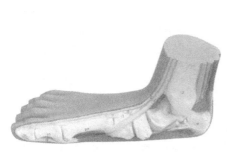

collapsed arch

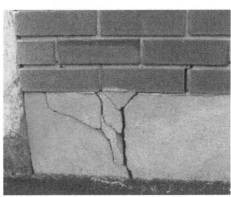

Cracked Foundation

Look at the difference in the foundation...

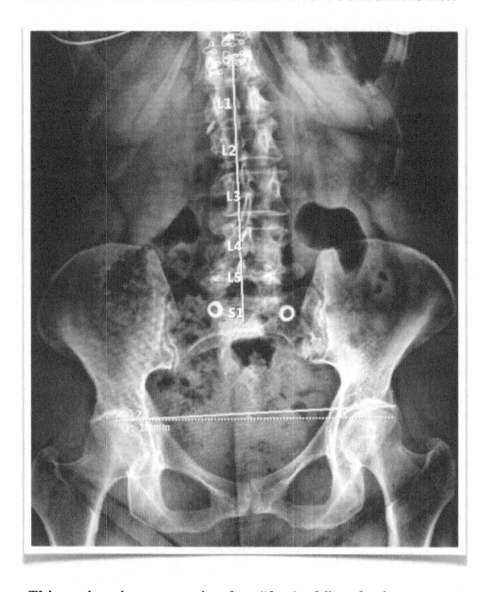

This patient is not wearing her "3- Arch" orthotics.

Notice how much straighter her spine is on the next page.

Also, look how much more level her pelvis is on the next page.

when "3-Arch" orthotics are in her shoes!

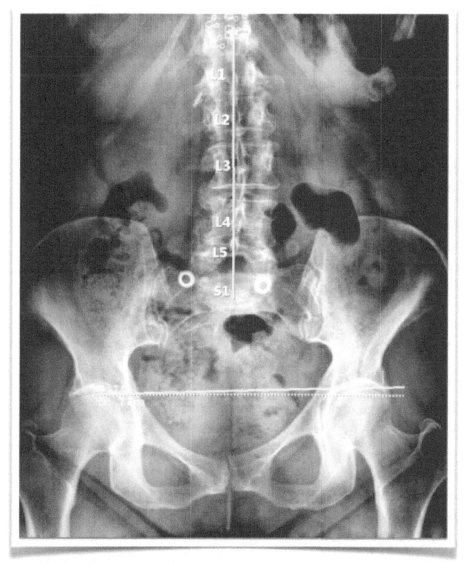

Straighter alignment, and a more level pelvis.

This is why I examine my patient's arches and only stabilize them with a "3-Arch" orthotic.

Case Study #1

Fallen arch leads to scheduled surgery!

A patient consulted to me last year about her lower back and left knee pain. She said she was scheduled for a knee replacement in October, which at the time, was just two months away.

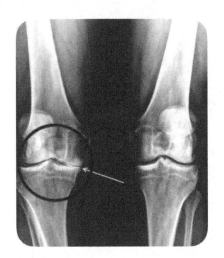

See how the cartilage in her left knee has grinded down.

When her arch collapsed it misaligned her tibia (leg bone) causing extra stress on her knee joint.

It probably took twenty plus years to wear out the cartilage.

The laser image of her feet showed both feet to be severely pronated, especially the left foot (see below).

See how her left arch has less contact with the surface than her right does.

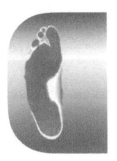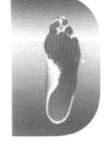

Left   **Right**

I ordered her orthotics and adjusted her lower spine and knee for one month with my computerized adjusting instrument. These adjustments helped de-compress and align both her lumbar spine and her knee joint. The orthotic helped to re-align her arches and removed the forces that were transferring up to her knee and back.

After two weeks she said that both her back and knee pain had decreased by almost 50%, and by the end of the 30-day window, her knee was at 95% efficiency. No knee replacement necessary!

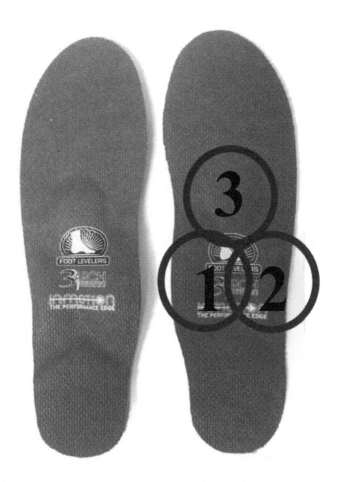

"3-Arch" orthotics I prescribed for her.

Case #2

The Boots don't lie!

Tom, who has been maintaining his lumbar spine with my clinic for about 2 years, told me his left knee hurt and had no idea why it was painful. He said he did not do anything he knew of to injure it.

I learned in chiropractic school that it is wise to x-ray the point of pain to be safe. As it turned out his left knee looked normal on x-ray.

Knees look normal,

but boots did not!

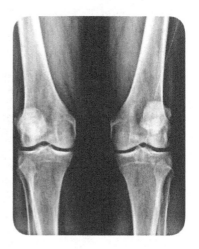

I had him take his shoes off and sure enough his left arch had fallen. I looked at the bottom of his work boots and they pretty well told the story (see next picture). I could clearly see the difference in the tread on his Red Wings!

The left back of the heal had worn at twice the rate because of the added stress on it from his fallen arch. I prescribed him "3-Arch" orthotics and on his next visit one month later, he said his knee pain was gone.

Normal wear   Worn out side

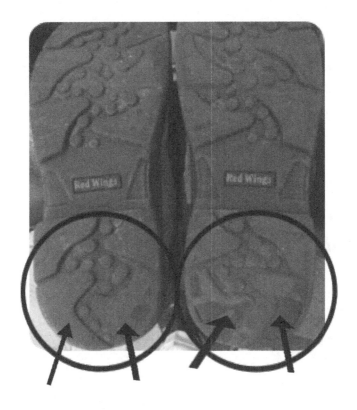

Outer arrows show how the heal of his left shoe is worn out.

Inner arrows show how those 3 round pads are completely gone on the left shoe!

Looking at the bottoms of your shoes may give you a clue as to whether or not you need to support your arches better.

Case #3

Achilles rupture hits home!

In 2018 my brother, David, was playing pickle ball and when he accelerated to make a play, he ruptured his Achilles tendon. He had surgery and was out of commission for the better part of four months.

This is a ruptured Achilles tendon!

Surgery is the next step!

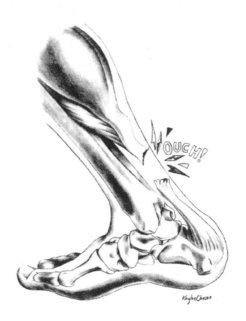

A few months after he had recovered, I felt a strain on my right Achilles tendon while I was on a stair stepper at the gym. I was very concerned because many times weaknesses can run in families, so I was overly cautious and decided to curtail my running and stair stepping for a week. To my surprise, I continued to have pain in the tendon.

A light then went off in my head to transfer my orthotics into my Brooks running shoes, as I have a slight pronation. Even though, Brooks have always been a great shoe to handle my pronation, I thought a better support may be necessary.

I transferred my "In Motion" orthotics into my Brooks shoes and proceeded to run a mile on my treadmill and there was absolutely no pain. This told me that the pronation was in fact causing a strain on my Achilles!

Since then I got a second pair, so I have them in both pairs of shoes.

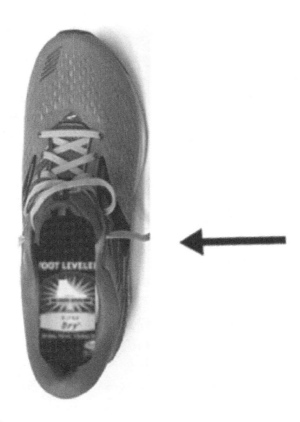

These re-aligned my Achilles tendon!

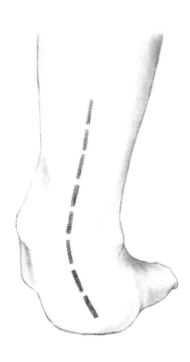

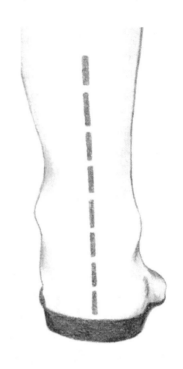

Pronated   *"3-Arch" orthotic*

Knee replacement surgery can be avoided many times with proper orthotics and knee adjustments!

I have had countless patients consult me about knee pain. An x-ray of the knee is a quick way to tell if someone is on the way to a knee replacement. Some of these patients have been scheduled for a replacement and we were able to cancel it because I put the patient in orthotics and adjusted their knee (See Case #1). This is a nasty surgery which requires long periods of rehabilitation **(see next page).**

$50,000 knee replacement or $295 for a "3-Arch" orthotic?

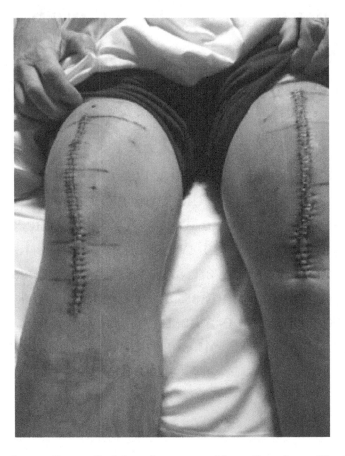

A patient shared this picture of her husband's knees, following his double knee replacement.

Look at those scars!

The cost of a single knee replacement with rehab is approximately $50,000!

The life of the replacement is around 18 years.

$100,000 lumbar fusion or $295 for a "3-Arch" orthotic?

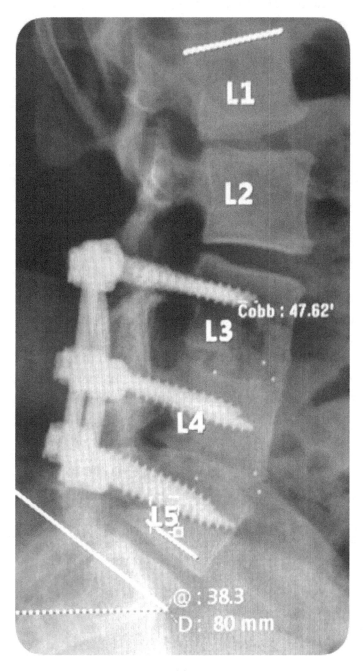

Take Home Message

✓ I think the arches of the feet are one of the two most overlooked areas (sacroiliac joint being the other), when trying to find the root cause of back pain.

I have consulted with many patients who have had steroid injections and some that even had surgery. Many of these same patients that had no relief from their pain had, in fact, a collapsed arch that was never addressed.

✓ I would estimate that one in five of my patients with a fallen arch, (that also had a previous history of taking steroid shots or had back surgery), had their pain reduced, by simply wearing orthotics.

✓ Fallen arches may lead to wear and tear on the lumbar spine and knee cartilage, which may ultimately lead to a fusion surgery and or a knee replacement.

✓ An orthotic will raise the fallen arch and help to eliminate knee joint destruction. This may solve not only unexplained knee pain, but also hard to resolve back pain.

✓ My favorite orthotic is: Foot Levelers because they are made from a laser image which is accurate up to 1 micron and <u>support all 3 arches</u>.

STEP 4

"Schultzing"

Walking is the best possible exercise.
Habituate yourself to walk very far.
-Thomas Jefferson

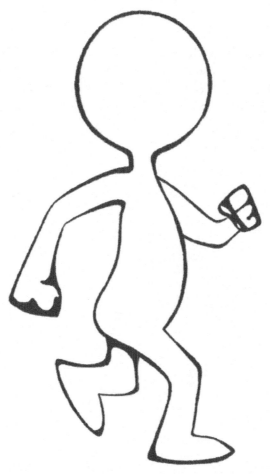

Kaylee Cheser

Did he just say walking?

In 1995, I went to a spine conference in New York, and the final speaker on stage that weekend was some award-winning German, PhD, orthopedist. His curriculum vitae was long and nothing short of amazing, but like many people with an exhaustive list of credentials, he was missing something. That something was the gift of keeping people or at least me awake, because he had me nodding off in what seemed like a New York minute.

So here I was, in a room filled with hundreds of well, how shall I say it? "real doctors", like neurosurgeons and orthopedic surgeons, and I think I must have been the only chiropractor there, and I was sleeping!

I suddenly woke up as I heard the words from the lecturer's mouth that he knows the very best exercise for back problems. It was as if I was back in high school daydreaming and everything the teacher said was being drowned out, until she said, "this is going to be on the test!"

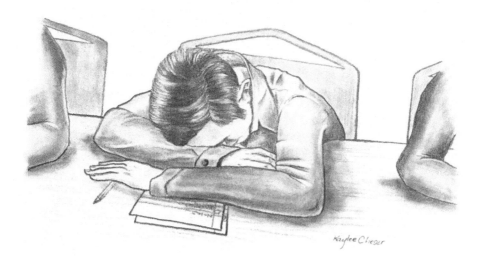

"Be quiet, the chiropractor is asleep."

PHd, Gives Best Exercise for the Back: Walking!

Did this PhD just say, "the one, very best exercise"? He did! He was going to answer a question that I had myself, for some time. Then he said it. It was WALKING. I was shocked, thinking "please tell me I did not spend $1,500 for this conference, plus nearly another $1,200 for an overpriced New York hotel room (which by the way, did not even offer free bottled water), only to hear that walking is the best exercise for the spine. That sounded way too simple!"

In fact, I was more than halfway surprised that this speaker from Germany, did not try to rename this simple exercise of walking after himself, calling it *"Schultzing"* or something, since orthopedists have been known to attach their names to tests and procedures.

Anyway, as boring as I thought he was, I was glad I invested my time at this conference because ever since then, walking has been my "go-to exercise" for my patients with back pain! (1)

Fitbit Craze!

A few years ago, my sister, Karen, told me that she bought an advanced tracking device called a Fitbit, and had been logging in 10,000 steps a day. She said her Fitbit helped her to stay on course to walk this many steps every day!

She demonstrated her device to me, and I was so impressed with the simplicity of it, that I got one for me and my wife.

Me with my sister, Karen.

If I ever need something stronger than mediocre advice, outside of my wife, Karen is my go to!

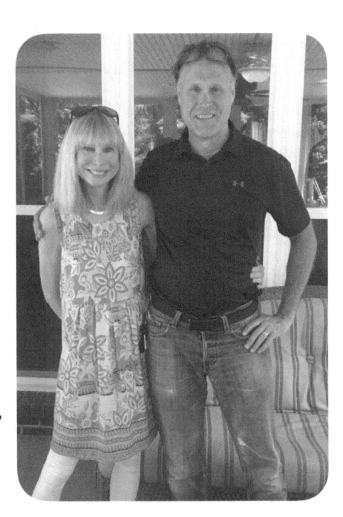

10,000 steps a day was first popularized by Japanese pedometers in the 1960s under the name "manpo-kei," which means "10,000 steps meter", according to UC Davis Integrative Medicine.

The Fitbit craze, I believe, is one of the best things to ever come about in the fitness era. I have seen people that never considered walking for exercise that are now trekking 3 to 4 miles every day. How cool is that?

I have bought a few Fitbit trackers. I kept getting the more and more expensive models, because I thought I would like all the additional bells and whistles. Having done this, I can tell you that in the end, my favorite one turned out to be the very first one I purchased. The simpler, lesser expensive model was just as efficient and easier to use. So, if you are so inclined to purchase one, I would try that one first, and with the extra money you save by not buying the premium tracker, you can put it towards a good pair of shoes, which I will address at the end of this chapter.

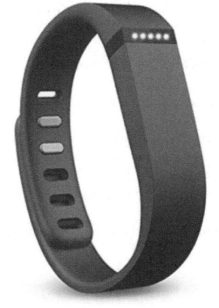

Dr. G's favorite Fitbit.

Simple!

Benefits of Walking

Below are just some of these benefits. (2)

1. Improves blood pressure

2. Improves blood sugar levels

3. Reduces the risk of coronary artery disease

4. Maintains body weight and lowers risk of obesity

5. Reduces the risk of breast and colon cancer

6. Enhances mental well-being

7. Reduces the risk of type 2 diabetes

8. Improves blood lipid profile

9. Decreases the risk of stroke by 20-40% (reported by research at the University of Bolder Colorado and the University of Tennessee)

10. Reduces risk of osteoporosis

11. Increases your creativity

12. Strengthens your secondary circulatory system, by increasing blood circulation from the leg muscles working more

13. Reduces the chances of varicose veins

14. Improves gastric mobility making you more regular

And according to Dr. Joseph Mercola's research, bare foot walking improves:

15. sleep disturbances; including sleep apnea

16. PMS

17. immune system activity and response

18. asthmatic and respiratory disorders

19. energy levels

20. rheumatoid arthritis

21. stress

22. fasting glucose levels.

In addition,...

...Dr. Joseph Mercola, a doctor of Osteopathy and New York Times best-selling author, reports that regular walking has been found to trigger an anti-aging process and help repair old DNA. If you want to add seven years to your lifespan, Mercola notes to set aside 20-25 minutes for a daily walk! **(1)**

"If you look at it, if everyone did just 10,000 steps a day in America we would probably decrease the healthcare budget by $500 billion a year. This shows how few people actually walk, and it also shows the price tag of chronic illnesses like diabetes, metabolic syndromes and heart disease," according to Michael Roizen a physician and chief wellness officer at the Cleveland Clinic.

Fortune 500 Companies are Getting in the Act!

The benefits involved with walking is prompting Fortune 500 companies to hand out fitness-based incentives. For example, employees participating in "United Healthcare Motion" can earn an additional $1.25 each day for reaching 10,000 steps over the course of 24 hours.

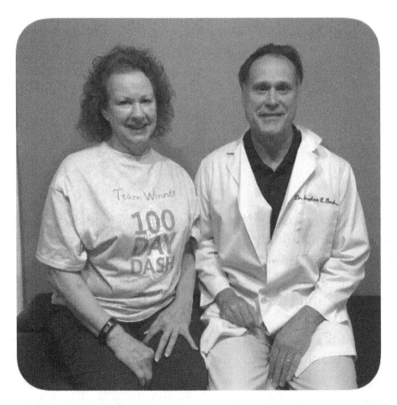

Diana is averaging over 10,000 steps a day and receiving incentives from her company!

Now that is impressive!

Walking: 6 Benefits for a Healthier Back!

#1 Strengthens Core

Walking **(1)** *strengthens the core* (3) as well as muscles in the legs and hips. I discussed this benefit at length in Chapter 3. In short, a good core acts as an armor of protection for the spine.

#2 Increases Stability of the Spine

Walking **(2)** *increases the stability of the spine* (4), meaning it promotes normal movement of the spinal bones. When someone sits on their rusty-dusty all day, the bones of the spine may:

1. jam-up or get sticky, this leads to
2. abnormal movement, causing
3. early degeneration to the disc, which may lead to
4. disc bulges, herniations, and potential
5. disc collapse.

In addition, abnormal movement can cause inflammation, which equals more Ibuprofen and stomach ulcers. This is the collateral damage that can take place when you make the decision to sit instead of move.

#3 Increases Blood Circulation

An advantage from walking is that the movement **(3)** *causes strong blood circulation* (5), thus pumping vital nutrients into soft tissues (muscles, ligaments and tendons). It helps drain any toxins as well.

#4 *Improves Flexibility and Posture*

Walking **(4)** *improves flexibility and posture* (6). The benefit from this is that the more range you have to bend and twist, the more likely your spinal muscles will have some give to them. So, when you are performing an awkward move, such as lifting a piece of furniture or reaching into the back seat of your car, your chances of injury are lessened.

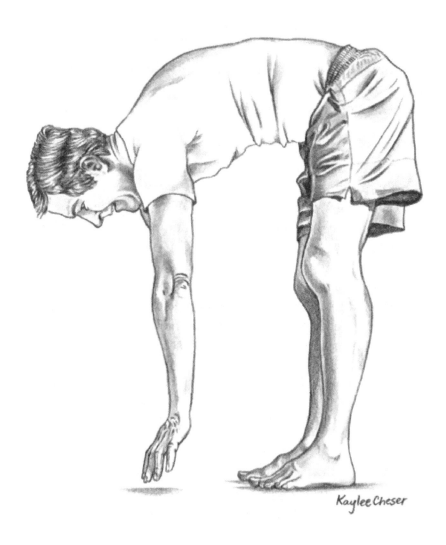

Kaylee Cheser

#5 *Strengthens Bones*

Increased amounts of walking will **(5)** *strengthen bones and reduces bone density loss*. (7) This is a naturally effective way to keep stress on your bones. Unfortunately, as we get older many people want to relax and not be as active, when in fact that is the very best time to engage in some physical activity. This lack of stress on the spine, increases the risk of spinal compression fractures.

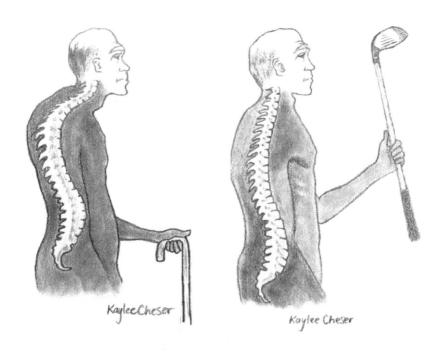

When you see elderly people that are hunched over to a point of looking uncomfortable, it is usually because they have multiple compression fractures. Compare them to the person who is 80-years old who is golfing and playing tennis. They probably don't have any fractures because they made better health care decisions, like walking!

#6 *Weight Loss*

One major benefit of walking is **(6)** ***increased weight loss***, (8) which in turn will decrease spinal pain. The more someone weighs, the more stress is received by the joints of the spine. This leads to an unstable spine with inflammation. Of concern to me, is the younger generations that are sitting all day at school followed by even more hours sitting and playing video games at home.

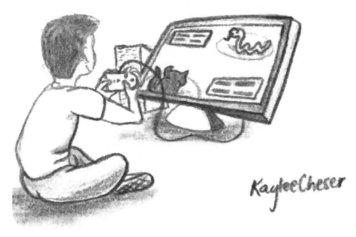

KayleeCheser

While they are young now and may think they're getting away with it, they will likely suffer down the road and regret the harm they inflicted in their youth.

As a side note: when I was in grade school, there was only one guy in our class that was overweight. Today, it is not uncommon to see a half-dozen children in one class that are substantially overweight. I would encourage the parents of these children for them to set the technology down, get out of the house, and get active!

If this exhaustive list has convinced you to get out there and walk, then there are a few things I would suggest you do first.

Find a Good Pair of Walking Shoes!

Investing in shoes is just as important as spending money on a mattress (Chapter 7). I would go to a reputable running store to buy walking or running shoes.

Thirty years ago, I went to the Ken Combs Running Store in Louisville, where I was surprised to be waited on by a University of Louisville cross country runner. How cool is that! I told him that I kept wearing out the ball of my right shoe and he had me walk and run down the side walk.

He thought because of the way my right foot had a slight pronation, that the Brooks shoes would be the best shoe for me. Ever since then, I always purchase shoes from a specialized store because of the people who work there. Amazon has a great delivery system, but with something as important as shoes, I just as soon go to a professional.

Dr. G's favorite shoe

Brooks Adrenaline GTS 19

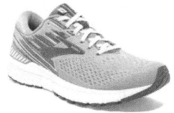

I would consider an insert if you are a pronator (one with a fallen arch). You can get good orthotics for walking/running shoes for about $40 (Powerstep-Pinnacle). I recommend these because they have firmer arches, which will offer you better support. If you are not sure if you pronate, the people that work at the running store can tell you.

If it hurts your back to walk, consider getting on a treadmill and holding on to the rails. This will become more like aquatic walking, taking a lot of the stress off of the lower spine. This way, you don't have to find a pool or have to put on a swimsuit in the winter, or for that matter, maybe not at all.

Good Tip from Dr. G

If you decide to use the treadmill for walking, you may want to adjust the incline. If you have a:

> ➤ *disc problem (hurts to sit)*-walk flat or at a decline.
> ➤ *spinal stenosis (hurts to stand)*- walk at an incline.

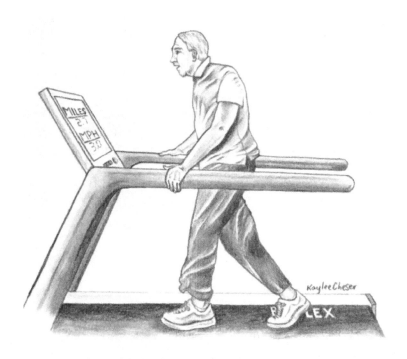

If your back hurts more to stand, merely adjust the incline to 1.

This is an easy way to take stress off your spine!

Take Home Message

✓ Walking is the very best exercise for your back. Walking is easy to do and just fun enough to look forward to doing every day. This enhances the likelihood of good follow through!

✓ The Fitbit is a great tracking device. I like the bare bones Fitbit the most. This device helps keep track of your steps every day without you having to think much. 10,000 steps are a great daily goal!

✓ Some benefits of walking include: strengthening the core, increasing stability of the spine, increasing blood flow, increasing flexibility, strengthens the bones, and helps to lose weight. All these are helpful towards a strong pain-free back!

✓ My favorite walking shoe is *Brooks Adrenaline GTS 19.*

STEP 5

Posture:

The Window to Your Spine!

Never bend your head. Always hold it high.
Look the world straight in the eye.
-Helen Keller

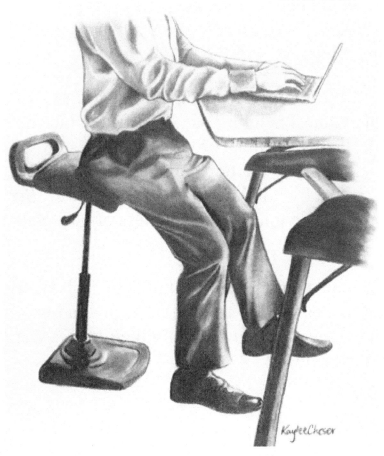

The Best Spine in Louisville!

In 1999, I had this "bright idea" about having a "Best Spine in Louisville" contest. I had an old, high mileage Mercedes Benz sitting in my garage that I never drove. My plan was to run an advertisement, have contestants come to my office, get some x-rays, and try to win the car. Great idea, right?

Wrong! The chiropractic board did not share the same enthusiasm as I did. They thought by me doing this, I would be radiating half of Louisville unnecessarily. So, I had to drop yet another one of my great ideas!

I got this thought from a picture that I saw of a posture contest held in 1956, in Chicago (see next page). Back then, the chiropractic profession was just getting some traction and a few chiropractors thought that by holding a *"Correct Posture" Beauty Contest*, they could raise awareness of our relatively new profession.

The contest included a plumb line analysis for overall balance and a front view X-ray that was taken to determine how straight their spines were (see next page).

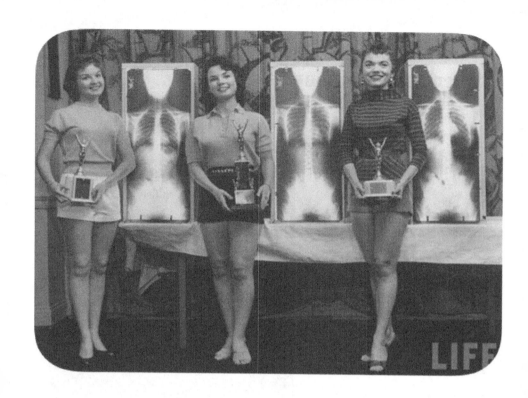

"Correct Posture" Beauty Contest.

This was held in 1956 in Chicago.

The one in the middle was the winner.

Her x-ray looks pretty straight to me!

When I examine a patient, I assess two different alignments of the spine.

1. <u>Straightness</u> (from a frontal view).

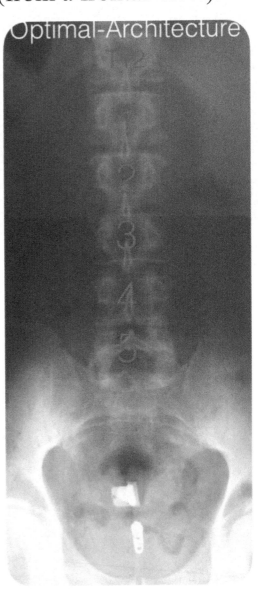

I am proud to say that this is my spine!

Nice and straight from the front!

2. <u>Angles</u> of the spine (side view)

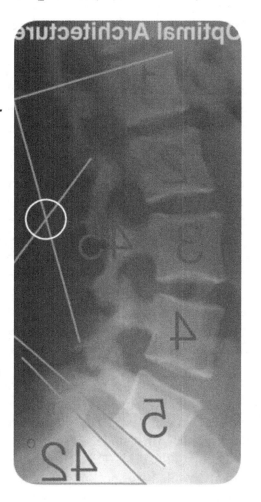

Notice the perfect 45-degree angle of the lower back.

The discs are thick.

This is great posture and I wish this x-ray were mine, also!

Oops! I just coveted thy neighbor's spine!

Good posture is crucial for the health of your back. Focusing on improving it brings forth many benefits to both your spine and discs. A healthier posture will strengthen your chances of escaping chronic back pain!

So how can we train our spines to have great posture? This involves how you sit, stand, and sleep. <u>Sitting and standing</u> is what the rest of this chapter is about; the sleeping part will be covered more in Chapter 7.

129

Big 8 accounting firm went cheap on the chairs!

I had a part-time, after school job for the tax season in 1979. The company I was working for was one of the "Big 8" accounting firms. Big 8 means it was one of the eight largest firms in the nation. Today, after all the mergers and acquisitions, they are one of the "Big 4".

National accounting firms at that time, spared no expense! Everything was the best of the best. Their building was magnificent, and most things inside were nothing less than pristine because impressing clients was their priority. They had the top of the line, *IBM Selectrics*. You remember, the ones with the "golf ball" heads. Back in the 1970's, these were the game changers in typewriter space.

All the Partners of the firm had fancy offices with big windows overlooking downtown Louisville. They all sat at big wooden desks with high back swivel chairs. This way anyone that walked by their office, including me, thought that they really had it going on!

Okay, now let's talk about what my "office" of a space looked like. Me and my buddy, Jim Morris, also from Bellarmine College, sat at these heavy metal desks. The chairs were these heavy clunkers, that looked like late fifty models. In fact, my arm rests on these banged into the top of the desk. This left me reaching, and hunched over all afternoon, while I was pecking away at my Toshiba 10 key calculator.

I still clearly recall, having to get up and walk around the office multiple times to stretch out my neck and back because they were so tight from sitting at an angle all day.

I thought this kind of pain was only reserved for people that worked on their feet all day at Ford or something, not a Big 8 accounting firm of all places!

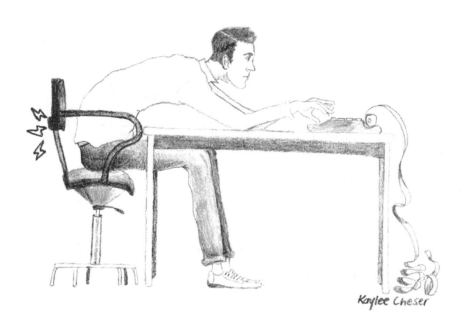

Kaylee Cheser

So why did the big green clunker cause my back to hurt so much?

A sitting, bent forward posture actually poses the second highest intradiscal pressure to be exerted on the spine (407 Pounds!!!). (1)

When I found out 10 years later how much I had been smashing the insides of my disc, I felt like the poor guy who unknowingly, was working in a room with asbestos falling out of the ceilings. In fact, I believe that chair could have set up my back to get injured a year later.

High intradiscal pressures is what initiates ***disc degeneration, bulging, and herniations***.

My experience at the accounting firm, made me want to kick off this chapter with ***intradiscal pressures*** of each postural position. (2)

Intradiscal Pressures

Pounds of pressure on the L5-S1 Disc.

(small of the back = L5-S1)

1. Laying down

This exhibits the least amount of intradiscal pressure. Because of this, laying supine is your best bet for taking stress off your low back (3).

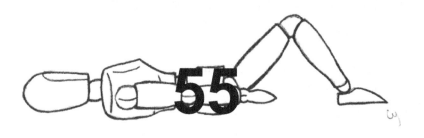

55 pounds (least amount of intradiscal pressure)

2. Standing

Standing as a whole, causes the second highest pounds of force to be exerted on the discs. Amounts of it vary: (4)

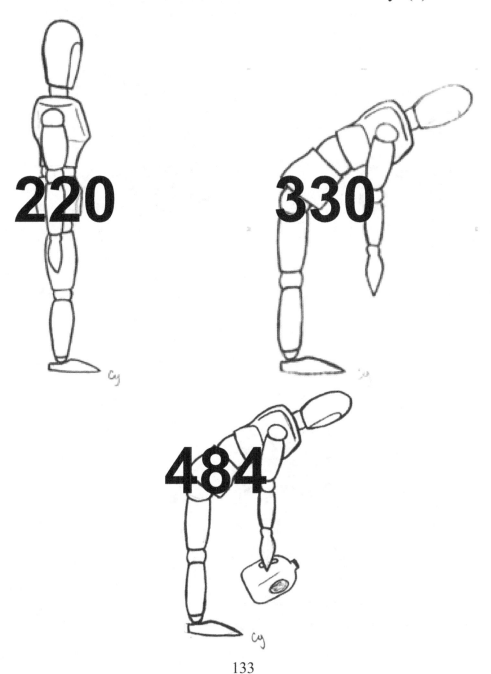

Sitting

This position causes overall, the **highest intradiscal pressures**! (5)

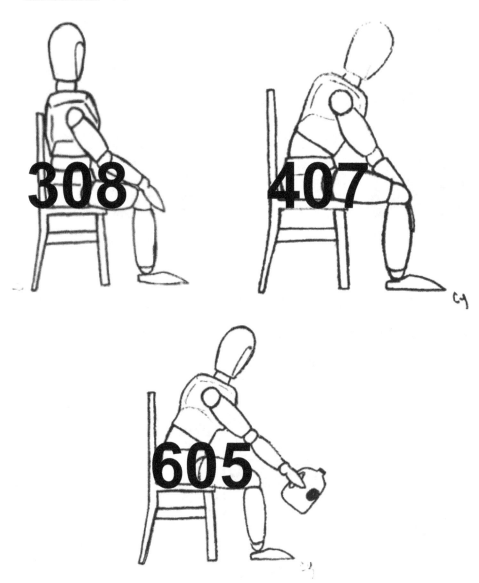

As we look at the different postures in this chapter, you will probably want to refer to this list.

Sitting is the "New Smoking"

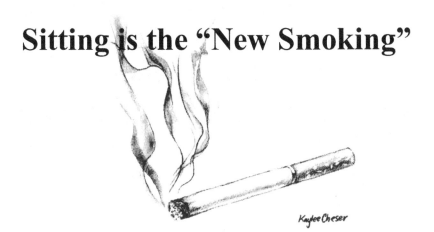

Kaylee Cheser

More than half of American back pain cases are from desk workers!

Back pain is no longer reserved for those who spend the majority of the day on their feet. Cases in one study proved that 54% of Americans experiencing pain spent most of their workday <u>sitting</u>. (6)

Research reveals that after a mere 20 minutes, the typical desk worker's postural muscles will start to fatigue, (7) resulting in the shoulders rounding, the neck leaning forward, and the low back stretching. This change of posture puts abnormal stress on the joints of the skeletal system. This can lead to poor spinal alignment, increased intradiscal pressure, and premature disc degeneration.

In addition, this constant pressure on the disc from sitting, can cause migration of the jelly material in the inner core of the disc, towards the spinal canal (slipped disc). This has the possibility of leading to a herniation.

Americans are sitting an average of 12-13 hours a day! You have got to be kidding me!

USA TODAY **I** FRIDAY, FEBRUARY 15, 2019 **I** 5B

Ergonomics important for heavy digital users

Marc Saltzman
Special to USA TODAY

Quickly, calculate how much time you spend in front of digital devices, such as computers, tablets, and smartphones. Be honest.

According to a recent Nielsen report, American adults spend about 11 hours per day on technology – that's about two-thirds of the time we're awake – and the number climbs higher for those who work in front of a monitor at the office. Americans now are sitting an average of 12 to 13 hours a day, says Ergotron, a manufacturer of office-related products.

If this sounds familiar, you bet your bitmaps there are health concerns with our sedentary work culture.

And so, take heed to these following "ergonomic" tips to healthier computer use, whether it's during your 9-to-5 work life, 5-to-9 downtime or both.

136

The 4th largest static pressure on the disc is sitting!

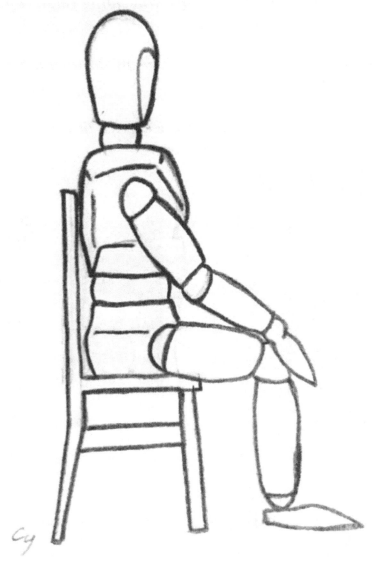

Prolonged times spent in this position acts as a dehydrator for the disc.

Look how the x-ray changes from sitting to standing!

Notice how the spine straightens with sitting versus the more natural arc with standing.

Sitting posture: The forces run directly through the discs (see arrows).

Standing posture: The forces are exerted through the back part of the spine (see arrows).

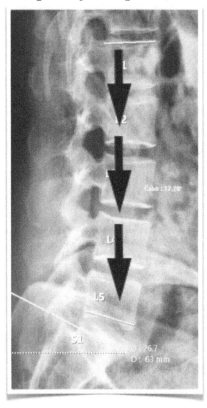 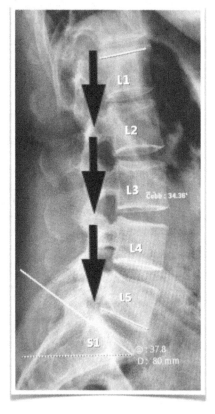

Sitting Posture   *Standing Posture*

Increases load on the disc   *Decreases load on the disc*

6-8 hours a day of sitting may take you from a great disc to a bulging disc!

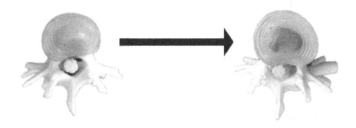

Poor work place posture causes increased forces primarily in the upper neck, lower neck, and the lower back.

Just imagine, if you continued to hold this position for hours at a time, with poor ergonomic furniture, these abnormal stresses would be even more magnified.

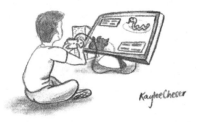

Even worse than that, are the school-age children that sit in class all day and come home only to play video games for hours upon hours. If that is not bad enough, they usually sit in the worst posture imaginable, sitting and leaning forward (highest intradiscal pressure).

For parents to see and know this information, it is no different than exposing young, innocent children to second hand smoke. It is no wonder that I am getting more and more calls from mothers, scheduling their children because their neck and back hurt.

2 Postural Cases

Postural Case #1

A few years ago, a surgical assistant consulted with me about headaches that she was experiencing on a daily basis.

An x-ray of the side of her neck showed that it was rounded forward (reversed arc compared to the normal arc), reflecting her typical work posture. Since she had been working in this profession over ten years, her spine, more than likely, had reshaped to that position. It turned out that this bad alignment is what had led to her headaches.

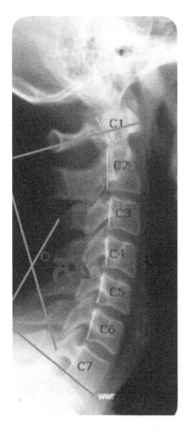 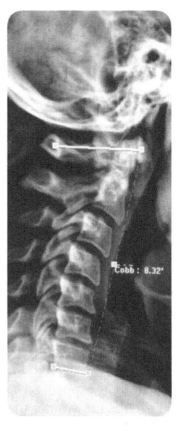

normal arc   *reversed arc-not good!*

140

- *You can easily see that her neck has lost its normal posture.*

- *This posture stretches the spinal cord and leads to bone and disc deformation.*

- *This leads to headaches and neck problems.*

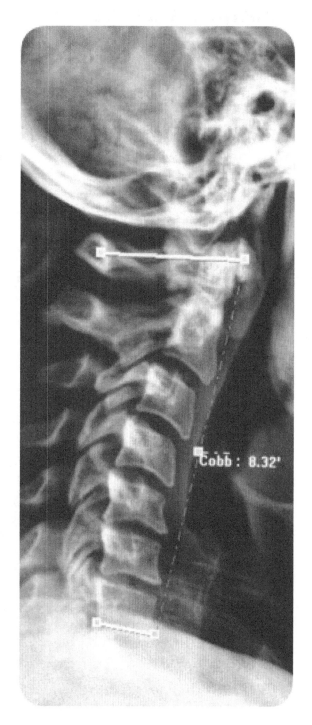

Postural Case #2

A 42-year-old female came to my office for headaches and neck pain. Her occupation was in office sales, so it was not uncommon for her to be on the phone for lengths of time. Her x-ray revealed a tilt to the right, which was the exact side that she had cradled her phone to. Eventually her spine, more than likely, aligned into that position.

This posture is prone to put abnormal stress on the lower discs in the neck.

This can lead to disc degeneration and disc bulges!

Common symptoms from this are:

✓ *neck pain,*
✓ *numbness and tingling into the arm and hand*
✓ *headaches!*

If you adopt a bad posture, it may permanently alter your spine.

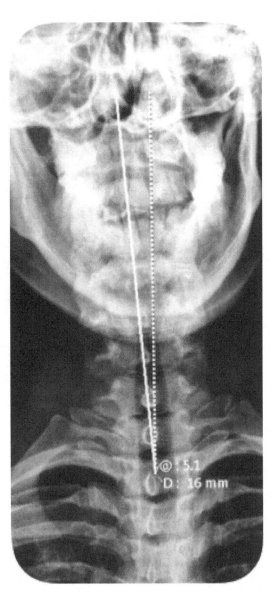

142

7 Ideas for Better Posture and Less Intradiscal Pressure

#1 Adjustable chair

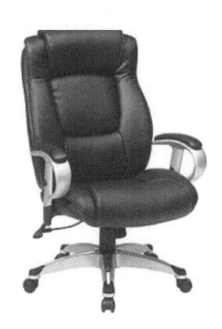

Basic adjustable, run of the mill, chair from an office supply store

Either way you look at it, sitting is sitting, and it is not good to do all day. This sitting erect posture, carries the third most intradiscal pressure of all postures. (8) So, what are the very best chairs to sit in?

The best chairs are ones where the arm rests fit underneath their desk and are positioned where they are not jamming your arms into your shoulder sockets. Conversely, the arm rests should not be so low that your elbows cannot rest comfortably on them, as that can lead to neck strain.

A good chair also should allow your feet to touch the ground flat, with your hips at 90 degrees.

Since not all chairs are made for people that are 4'11" or 6'3",...

.....it is best to have chairs that have adjustable features that can accommodate each individual's correct posture. These chairs are more expensive, but with health in mind, are worth it.

Ergonomic chairs, while extremely efficient for the spine, can get pricey. I came across a company with the name of Human Solutions, where I found a chair called the Humanscale Freedom for a whopping $949. Are you kidding me?

Personally, I would start at a Staples or Office Depot, and see if there is one there that works for you. I have found that specialty stores are very expensive and are not always better.

Years ago, I found a chair for about $150 at Staples, that was a perfect fit for my height and was built well. It supported me well and as a result, I was totally comfortable no matter how long I was in it. In fact, I still have it today!

Great Tip:

Do not cross your legs when you sit. An instructor at Logan, Dr. Diamond, taught me that when you cross your legs in the sitting position, you can knock your pelvis right out of alignment.

Thank you, Doctor D!

#2 Exercise ball

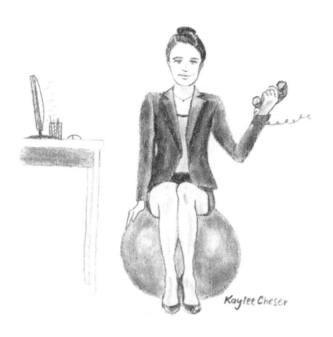

Kaylee Cheser

Another option is to sit on an exercise ball. I really like these for the multitude of benefits they provide, in addition they are fun!

In this posture, the pelvis is rocked gently forward, increasing the angle of the lumbar spine, which takes stress off the lower disc. This posture will also naturally shift the shoulders back.

Exercise balls are great for the abs, too. It forces you to balance yourself continually, so you are constantly activating all of your abdominal muscles.

You can purchase a great exercise ball for around $50, which is less than the cost of a gym membership!

#3 Varichair

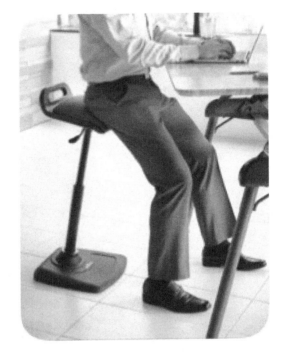

Great Chair!

The Varichair acts more like an exercise ball (without the ab benefit) in that you sit more on the edge of it, which takes stress off the discs, by transferring the load to the back of the spine. This chair can also be adjusted down to accommodate the regular desk.

Because the chair is a mixture of standing and sitting, you are essentially averaging two intradiscal pressures. Can you imagine how much more productive you could be, if you were not fatigued by having aches or pains?

I believe that for the benefit it offers to your spine, it is fairly priced at $195.

#4 Stand-up desks

A. Varidesk.

I prescribed my patient Rebecca, a Varidesk (see below)! They are advertised on TV and she told me they are every bit as good as advertised!

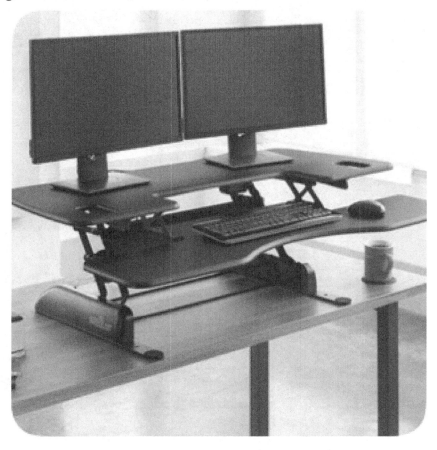

Now this is really cool!

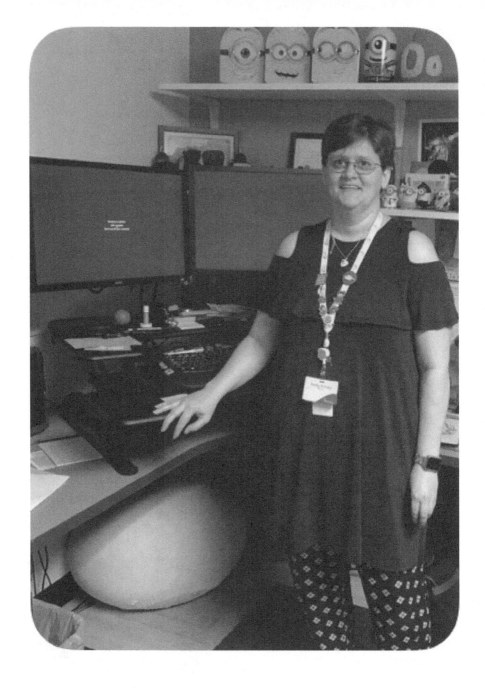

- *By switching to the Varidesk, Rebecca reduced her intradiscal pressure by 88 lbs.*

- *This helped to eliminate her back pain!*

B. Adjustable desks

A few years ago, I was the guest speaker at a Brown Foreman symposium. Before the lecture, Richard Wimsatt, their marketing chief, was kind enough to give his lifelong friend, a tour of the campus.

One of the many things that impressed me was how many of the workers had adjustable stand up desks. At Brown Foreman, the same desk may be used by multiple people, so they were constantly switching positions throughout the day. You can quickly grasp the benefit from being able to adjust the desk for someone who is 5'5" or 6'5".

I also like the Quick Pro 60 Butcher Block from Varidesk. I like its simplicity and it is so much better than sitting all day. This desk is $495.

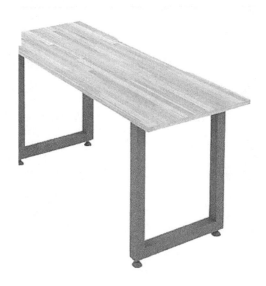

Simple, yet so practical!

I think stand up desks are definitely on an upward trend. Even though they may be considered an expensive upgrade, it is a lot less than the cost of an examination by an orthopedist or neurosurgeon. So, I say, if your company is open to this idea, I would consider asking them to purchase a stand-up desk for you.

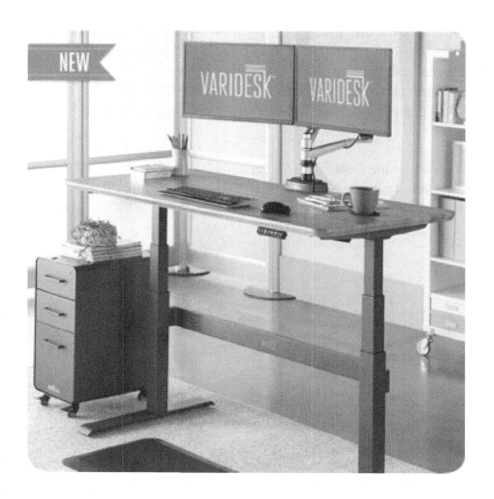

A very impressive set-up!

Sharon came to our clinic with chronic back pain.

Her disc at L5-S1 has visible degeneration.

I prescribed a stand-up desk for her to take stress off her bottom disc while she works.

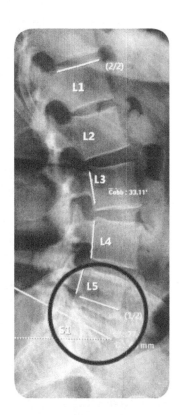

Her company invested in an adjustable stand-up desk.

She reduced her daily intradiscal pressure on her lower back by 88lbs. overnight!

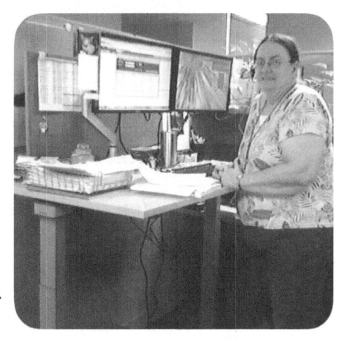

#5 Lumbar cushion

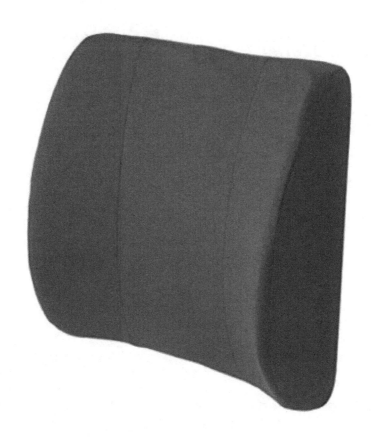

The Relax-A-Bac

- *Has a wooden lumbar support board and strap.*
- *Amazon.com sells these for $25, and trust me, that is a bargain!*

I have been using a lumbar cushion for many years. I was first turned on to these my very first semester in chiropractic school. I can still remember duct taping it to my chair in the perfect position, so it would not slide around.

Since I was sitting in class the first two years from 7A to 2P, I got a lot of use out of that thing. I used that same cushion all four years of school. It really saved my back!

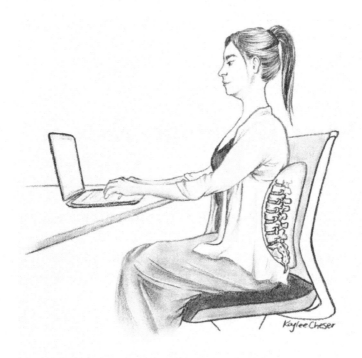

In the normal sitting position, the back flattens out and you will get hit with 400+ pounds of pressure. The benefit of using a lumbar cushion, is it causes the spine to return to the natural 45-degree arc, conforming to the natural curve. This way of sitting significantly reduces intradiscal pressure.

You guessed it. Lumbar cushions are like cars; you can spend a little or you can spend a lot.

The **Relax-A-Bac** lumbar cushion, unlike most, have a hard back to them which gives them more stability. I have turned many patients on to this model and they absolutely love them. I honestly believe, if every worker who sits for a living, would purchase a **Relax-A-Bac**, a whole lot of back pain would be eliminated in the United States of America!

Some chairs have built-in cushioning. I have found these not to be as beneficial as a specialized cushion. So, for about 25 bucks, you can add a lot of support and happiness to your lower spine.

#6 The "five-minute re-boot"

With all of the electronic gadgets flooding the market, find one that can alert you so that you can get up and move around every 30 minutes. There are Fitbit trackers and watches that you can set to vibrate on your wrist. The main thing is, you just have to get up, move, and give yourself a re-boot!

In fact, a study published in American College of Occupational and Environmental Medicine found that *switching between sitting and standing throughout the workday can lead to a 54% reduction in neck and back pain.*

#7 Postural exercises

I especially like these 5 exercises you can do right at your workplace:

1. Chest stretches.

Put your hands in the doorway and stretch out your chest. When you are working at your desk, your shoulders will rotate forward, and your chest will contract. This exercise will reverse this forward rotation, by stretching out your shoulders, chest/torso, waking it up. Not only does it do your torso a huge favor, but it feels great!

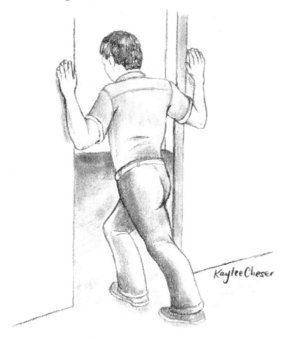

Do these: **5 times with a three second hold.**

As you do this a few times, you may want to go to 10!

2. Scapula pinches.

After sitting for a few hours, your upper back muscles stretch, and nothing feels better than to pinch your shoulder blades. These scapula pinches will reverse the effects of these stretched muscles.

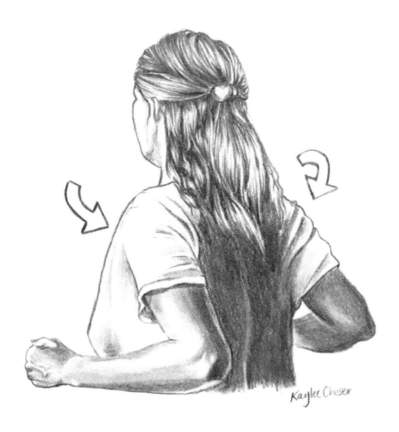

*The best way to do these, is to stand up and squeeze your blades together and **hold for 3 seconds**. Repeat ten times.*

3. Trap stretch.

When you sit a long time, the trapezius (trap) muscle tightens up on both sides around your lower neck, probably causing you to want someone to massage your neck and upper back. The next best thing to this, is to stretch your trap muscle.

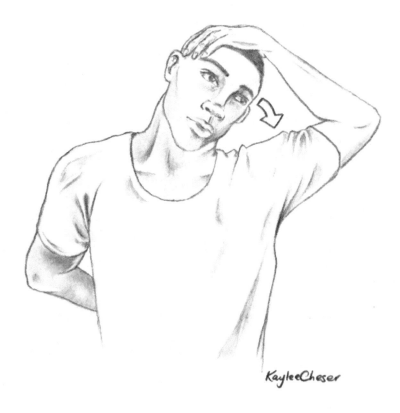

KayleeCheser

*Just put your hand over the top of your head and bend it to the side, **holding for 5 seconds,** and do the same for the opposite side. Do each side 3 times.*

4. Neck stretches.

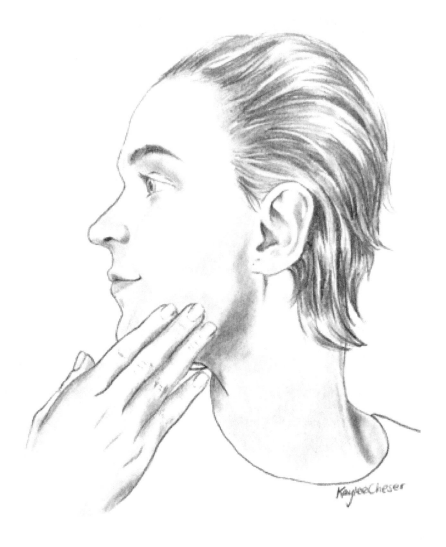

Rotate your head in six different directions (forward, backwards, side to side, and left to right) and **hold for 3 seconds**. This will stretch all the muscles that have shortened from fatigue.

5. Hip flexor stretch.

When you sit, the psoas muscle (pronounced "so-ass") becomes weakened and can lead to chronic back pain. Get on one knee with your hands on your hip and lean forward. The psoas muscle will stretch on the side where the knee is down.

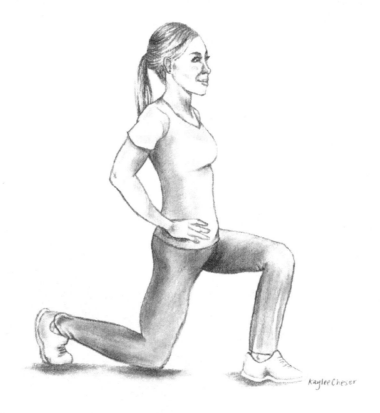

*Do these 5 times with each hip and **hold for 3 seconds**. This is especially important if you drive a lot of miles for a living.*

If you are short on time do three of the five. I am confident you can do all of these in five minutes.

Do those 5 exercises every day. You will feel more energetic and jazzed all day. This is better than drinking that fourth cup of coffee!

Posture Corrector

Recently, a patient returned to my office boasting about his posture corrector he bought from Amazon. I asked him if he could show it to me. Well, he proceeded to take his shirt off and there over his t-shirt, he had what looked like a black harness around his back. He showed me how he tightens it up and said that it pulled him back into better alignment. I have to admit that I thought it was a pretty impressive device.

That same day I ordered a posture corrector from Amazon for $21. For me having to bend over people all day it was too restrictive. However, if you have a desk job, I would definitely consider this posture corrector.

Posture Corrector.

"Ovation Home"

Purchase it from Amazon

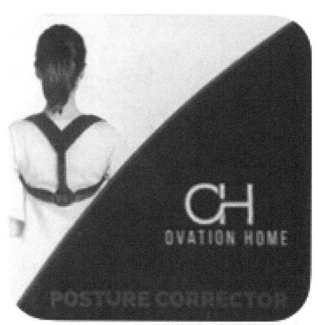

This will help you keep your shoulders back when sitting all day at work!

When you first start, I would recommend 20 minutes the first day and continue adding 20 minutes to an hour each day until you can go the whole day with it on.

As a side note when I was in 6th trimester in chiropractor school, Dr. Casper told us that if you listen closely to what the patient says, they will give you the answer. I have never forgotten that tip. This was just another example of another patient giving me another great idea!

Enjoy your "Posture Corrector"!

Bonus material

Good posture in the car

There are just a few angles and positions you need to know about when driving to keep the intradiscal pressure down.

Sitting position

Keep your thighs parallel in the seat. If your knees are bent at too much of an angle, it will cause additional stress on your lumbar discs. (Remember the 308 pounds of intradiscal pressure).

Seat back position-100 degrees

Tilt your seat back to about 100 degrees, just slightly leaning back past straight up and down. The more linear the seat, the more force pressing down on the discs.

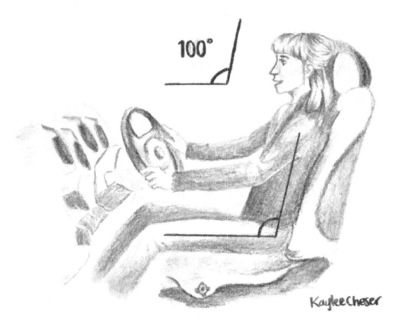

Lumbar cushion

If your car has an inflatable lumbar cushion, it will gently press on the small of your back to keep it in a favorable position. You will know when it is inflated properly, because it will feel natural for your back. This alleviates some of the stress off your discs when you are driving.

If you don't have a built-in cushion, then I would purchase a thin one advertised for a car (see the one below that is in my car). It should be thin enough that it does not move your head too far from the headrest as it will cause a larger, more serious whiplash, should you get rear-ended. I used to have one when I had my 1980 Honda Prelude.

This is a GREAT Lumbar cushion!!!

Dreamer Car
Auto Seat
Lumbar Support

From Amazon

$33.49

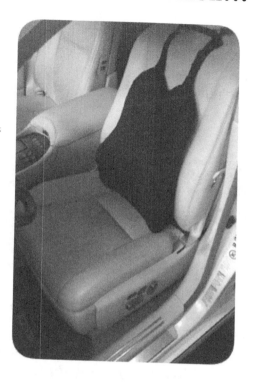

Made of
high density
memory foam

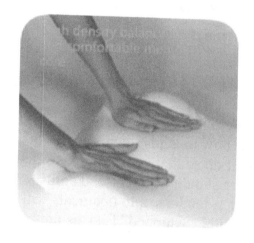

This is the one that Dr. G. has in his car!

Headrests

If you ever watched Perry Mason, you probably remember seeing his 1958 Cadillac convertible. Well, if you take a close look at the front seat of his car, you will see there is no headrest. It wasn't until the late 60's that these were introduced.

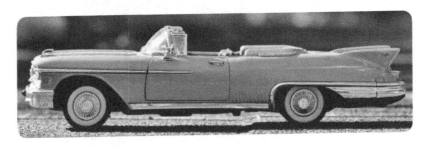

1958 Cadillac with no head restraints.

Until the late 60's there were no head restraints to keep the head from whipping right into the back seat, in a rear end collision!

More about headrests......

These are a great safety addition, and yet some drivers don't know how to adjust them. So, if you have never adjusted yours, raise it up so that your head hits squarely on the rest. This way, if there should be a rear-end collision, the damage to your neck muscles, tendons, and ligaments will be minimized, as your head will not be "whipped" back as far.

See how the back of the head hits squarely on the head rest.

This will prevent the head from whipping back, thus minimizing a neck injury!

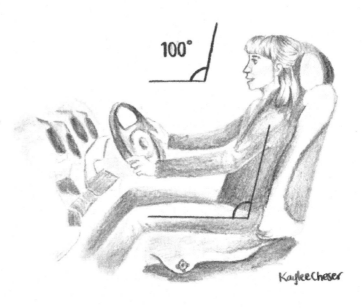

If the rest is set too low, your head could ramp up over it in a rear end collision, causing a more violent injury as there will be little to no protection. Then, you may find yourself looking up at the inside of an MRI tube!

Mirrors

Once you have your most fitting posture, set your mirrors. The mirrors will serve as a self-reminder for when you start to slouch because you will not be able to see properly out of them.

Stretching

I like to get out of my car every 100 miles just to stretch. As I mentioned earlier, if you drive a lot of miles for your job, you should definitely do the *psoas stretch*. This is a great exercise for those who spend an excessive amount of time in a sitting position.

Even the best of cars, for example a luxury Mercedes, still will subject you to whole body vibration. This vibration goes right through your spine, principally to your discs. So, leave a little earlier on those long road trips so that you can get out of your car a few more times.

Take Home Message

✓ Sitting in the workplace causes 54% of low back problems. **Sitting causes the most intradiscal pressure of all postures** (308 lbs.), followed by standing (220 lbs.). If a person sits on the job, they are increasing the pressure on the disc by 88 pounds, compared to when they stand.

✓ Increased intradiscal pressure increases the chances for disc bulges and disc herniations.

✓ The best way around this problem is to get a stand-up desk.

- My favorite stand-up desks are the **Varidesks**. These are priced fairly, and all my patients do nothing but rave about these.
- The particular desk I like the most is the desk top Varidesk which is priced at about $350.

✓ If you have a desk job, I recommend that about every couple hours do some **postural exercises** to take stress off your spine. The ones I outlined take less than 5 minutes.

✓ The **Relax-A-Bac** ($25) is my favorite lumbar cushion for the desk. The **Dreamer Car Auto Seat Lumbar Support** ($33.49) is my favorite lumbar cushion for the car. Both of these can be purchased on Amazon.com.

STEP 6

The Top 3 Mattresses...
...and Pillows!

When you lie down, you will not be afraid;
when you lie down, your sleep will be sweet.
-Proverbs 3:24

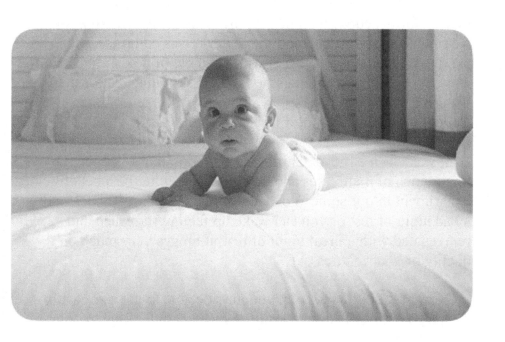

I learned from a juvenile delinquent about mattresses!

When I was a young boy, one of my all-time favorite fairy tales was *Goldilocks and The Three Bears*. As a 4-year old, I thought it was pretty comical how Goldilocks broke in the bears' home, ate their food, busted their chair, and slept in their beds.

At the time, I did not think of her as a rude, entitled little juvenile delinquent. My young mind was only able to process her as the harmless, lost little girl who just could not get comfortable in two of the beds, with the third one feeling just right! So, I learned at an innocent, youthful age, from a fairy tale, that not all beds are created equal.

By the time I turned twelve, our family had outgrown our modest three-bedroom home. So, my father built a room in the basement for my brother and me. After it was complete, my parents stocked our new room with a couple of box springs and mattresses. To make a long story short, I kept this bed for the better part of twenty years; I even took it with me to Logan College. It became a part of my life.

It was when I was in Chiropractic school, that I learned the importance of mattresses and how they can either be a benefit or a detriment to our spine. You can wake up with a stiff back and a bad night of rest or you can wake up feeling refreshed and rejuvenated with a great night of rest; it hinges very much on the quality of your mattress.

Now as a 20-30-year old, you may be able to get away with sleeping on a bad bed, like I did. As we get older, though, our spines are not as forgiving, and we need to get serious about what we are going to spend 30% of our lives laying on. (1)

Are You Sleeping in Good Alignment?

If you are sleeping on a mattress that is too soft or too hard, your spine could be out of alignment for the duration of six to eight hours. Now, a night or two of that in a bed out of town is not threatening to the wellness of your back, but if you do this night after night, year after year, your spine will more than likely, conform to the position you are sleeping in.

So, what does this mean for you? Let's say that mattress sag (an area of the mattress where the springs or coils have deformed) causes additional stresses on the bottom two spinal bones. If you lay on this for too many years, the disc in between them may get dehydrated, which is a precursor to degeneration.

As I mentioned in the anatomy chapter, a dried-up disc leads to bulging and herniations which can cause real pain!

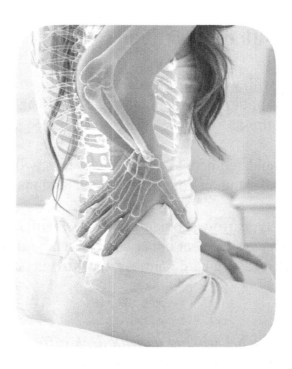

Beds Affect Alignment Differently

This bed was "too hard!"

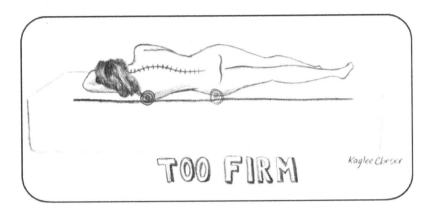

TOO FIRM

Kaylee Closer

Notice that a mattress that is <u>too firm</u> does not allow the pelvis to sink enough, which imbalances the hips, throwing the whole spine out of alignment for the entire night's sleep.

Challenges with different builds

- <u>Females with wider hips,</u> may cause even a greater distortion of the lumbar spine, as the pelvis sinks deeper in the mattress.

- <u>Wide shouldered</u> people, with smaller hips will generally experience shoulder compression on a hard mattress. (2)

- Conversely, <u>narrow shouldered</u> females, with larger hips will not have sufficient upper body weight to depress the shoulder area of a hard mattress, resulting in neck stiffness.

<u>Dr. G's Tip:</u> If you are waking up with neck stiffness every morning, it may not be a bad pillow, it may be your mattress.

This bed was "too soft!"

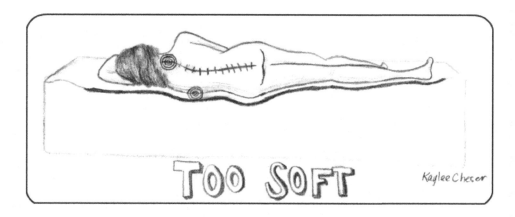

In this scenario, the pelvis sinks too much, again disrupting the alignment of the spine.

Not only do people using this type of mattress often wake up with a stiff spine, but just as detrimental, they may be robbed of a good night of sleep. Together, these will make for a bad day!

This bed feels "just right!"

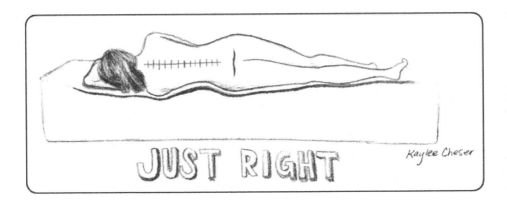

A great mattress should provide an environment in which the skeletal system is fully supported, while maintaining correct postural alignment.

You can see in the illustration above that the pelvis sinks enough so that it keeps the entire spine in proper alignment. This type of bed will afford people premium rest.

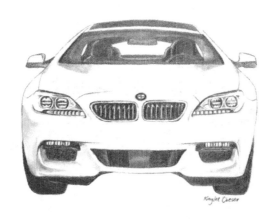

People invest 20-30 times more for a car than a good mattress!

On average, people spend 20-30 times more on a car than they do for a mattress. I realize a car is an absolute necessity for most people. Think about it. We are in our cars roughly one to two hours a day compared to a bed that we are in for six to eight hours a night. So, close to four times as long.

I really enjoy my job, and trust me, there is nothing better than to jump out of bed after a great night of sleep rather than dreading getting up. There is a direct correlation of when I wake up energized and comfortable, and how well my day goes. In contrast, when I don't have a good night of sleep, my day not only gets off to a rough start, but it often times does not finish strong. Big difference!

Would you want to let yourself fall victim to being uncomfortable and dragging for 365 days a year for years? Or would you be better served by getting a slightly less quality car and a higher quality mattress?

The worst mattress for the back!

The box spring and mattress

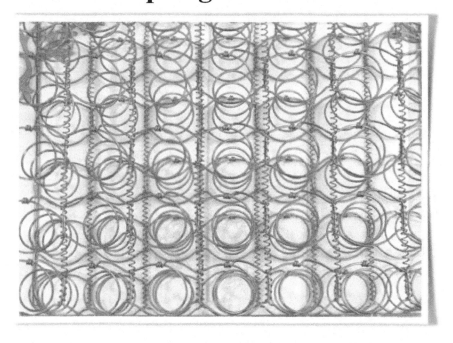

In an age with facial recognition, self-driving cars, and Smart TV's, box springs are considered old technology! They should have gone out in the 70's with the Pinto, the 8-track tape player, and platform shoes.

The only advantage I see, is the cost. You can buy a box spring and mattress today for a few hundred dollars. The consequence is, it is hard on your body as the springs are pushing and working against you all night. This may result in poor nights of sleep and if that is not bad enough, your back, more than likely, will be stiff in the morning.

In addition to possibly waking up stiff most mornings, spring mattresses needs to be turned over every three months. Flipping the mattress is necessary, because the weight of the body has been pushing on the same springs and over time they deform and cause mattress sag.

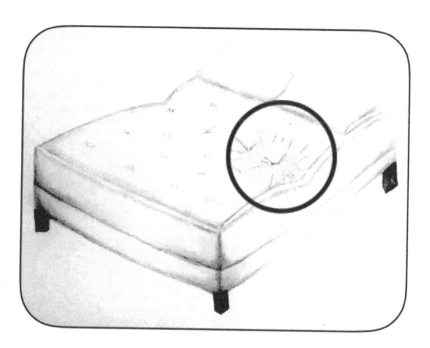

"Mattress Sag"

Rotating the mattress gives the springs a chance to regain their bounce and eliminate sag. The problem is, who on this planet rotates their bed every ninety days, except for people like my wife, Donna, and maybe her sister. When I had a spring mattress, I did not rotate it but one time, and this was on accident when I moved!

Make no mistake about it, if you want a mattress that will do more harm than good for your spine, and while getting a bad night of sleep to go along with it, I would highly recommend the box spring mattress.

Of course, there are exceptions to everything. For example, my friend's dad, drank a quart of whiskey a day until he was 94 and outlived three of his doctors!

G's
"Top 3"

If you are like me, you have probably slept in dozens of beds over your lifetime. I have slept in a few that I wanted to forget about (Motel 6) and then I have slept in some that I just could not get enough of.

There are dozens and dozens of mattresses on the market, and like most products, we know that much of the quality will depend on what the price tag is. For example, we know that $100 mattress will not be the same quality as a $900 mattress. But what about $800 versus $1,000 mattress, or $2,000 versus a $3,000 mattress?

This category of mattress ($1,000 and up) is a flooded market. There are dozens of brands out there fighting for your hard-earned money!

So, my "Top 3", is designed to help you to identify the good from the great even though there might not be a big difference in the price. I hope this helps you in some way!

So here is G's "Top 3" mattresses...

#3

Sleep Number

In 1996, I was laying on one of those fancy beds at the St. Matthews Mall, playing with the remote control. It was fun, changing the pressure of the air chamber, and feeling my spine raise up and down. To the salesman's delight, I stepped up that very same day, and purchased *The King Size Select Comfort.*

When the bed was delivered to my house, I again played with the sleep number, just as I had in the store. I blew it up and down and every which way. I probably did this for a full hour. Then, I found my sweet spot. 75 pounds was the magic number for me. It stayed on that exact number for 21 years! Compared to my old mattress, my night of sleep was like night and day.

Select Comfort developed the *Sleep Number Bed.* They are the only company that has the air chamber technology. The air chambers replaced the spring/coil technology. The two air chambers are encased with memory foam. There are multiple types of these beds and just like automobiles, their prices are determined by the thickness of the mattress and all the extra bells and whistles. *Sleep Number Bed* are referred to now as "Smart Beds" complete Sleep IQ technology! They even have an App that allows you to track your sleeping patterns. As of recent (2018), the **price ranges from $2,397 to $10,797**.

Their main benefit of the sleep number mattress is that you do not have springs, that over time will lose their elasticity and develop sag. The springs are replaced by air. Pretty slick idea!

Another benefit is that your spouse can set his or her side and you can set yours to your own comfort. I think that it is very handy if you are married, which is why I am placing this bed, in what is an over-flooded number of beds on the market, at number 3!

#2

Sealy Posturepedic

In 2010, I made a trip to Sea Island, Georgia. My good friend has a vacation home there and he invited me down for some golf and chill time. I was amazed at the scenery of this island, but nothing to me was more impressive than the beauty and awe of the Atlantic Ocean!

After 18 holes of golf and some sea food, I retired to the bedroom that I was to sleep in. I was taken aback when I woke up the next morning at how well I had slept. I did not remember sleeping like that for a long time.

So, being the sharp chiropractor that I am, when I got out of this amazing bed that morning, I pulled back the mattress covers to see what kind of bed it was that put me in such a deep sleep. The label read *"Sealy Posturepedic"*.

This mattress is a hybrid type mattress. A Hybrid Mattress is a cross between box springs and a foam mattress. It has a nice springy feel and may be easier to move around on, than a foam mattress. The top foam layer has a comfortable, plush feeling, not allowing you to feel any individual coils.

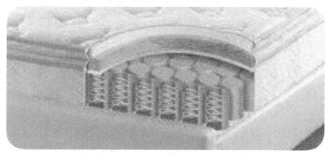

Memory foam with inner spring

179

Hybrids have a high coil count, which is more effective for weight distribution and support. This is a good transition mattress, because it retains the coils (for those spring-lovers) and will feel more luxurious because of the foam. Another benefit of the hybrid is, unlike springs, when you get up the whole bed does not shift around, decreasing the chances of waking up the other person

The larger gauged coils are in the center of the bed to accommodate the pelvis, as it is the heaviest part of the body (see below). You will find that the majority of the mattresses made today are Hybrids. Because of the coils, you will, more likely than not, need to replace your bed every 7-10 years because of mattress sag.

As you may have guessed, hybrid beds are priced between the box spring mattress and the 100% memory foam mattresses **(price range $790-$3,700)**. This is the sweet spot for most people's budgets.

Hidden inside the mattress are the coils.

Gray coils are heavier gauge, so the pelvis does not sink.

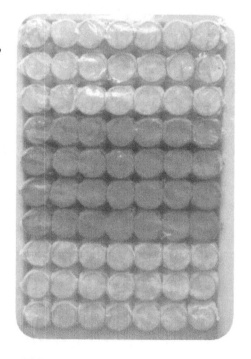

#1

Tempur-Pedic Mattress

There is Michael Jordon. And then, there is all the rest.

In 2017, I was getting married and we decided to invest in a new mattress. I already knew that I wanted to look at the Sealy mattress because of my experience in my friend's home at Sea Island. However, I also wanted to be fair to my wife and myself by going to some different stores and lay on some different mattresses to get a feel of what would be the best one for us jointly.

So, in June of 2017, I walked into a Sleep Outfitter Store and the associate there pointed me to the *Tempur-Pedic* line first. I had researched this bed a few years earlier when a patient had asked me about them. What I learned was that *Tempur-Pedic* was the first company to introduce memory foam. This was developed in the 1960's by NASA to protect astronauts from high impact landings.

Tempur-Pedic purchased the rights behind the memory foam (Temper Material) and developed a brand-new mattress category. The "Temper Material" sleep technology boasts the ability to self-adjust to your body's shape, weight, and temperature, distributing pressure for maximum support. Sounds pretty good to me!

Back to my encounter on the Tempur-Pedic...

I told the associate at Sleep Outfitters that I was most interested in sleeping on a "medium firm" mattress. I must have laid on 25 different beds before this, and as soon as my head fell back I told my wife, "this is it". Donna tested it out for herself, and she absolutely thought it was the most comfortable bed she ever laid on. It had the perfect feel.

Did I like the price tag? Not exactly. But after jotting down some numbers on the back of an envelope, I quickly figured out that if I kept the bed for 15 years or more, it was actually going to be no more expensive than any of the other mattresses, and I could get a much better quality of sleep. Since I have a history of hanging on to beds for a while, the 15 years was not going to be a problem.

Why do I Think I Get Such a Great Night of Sleep?

1. Density

The denser foam makes for a more relaxing experience.

2. Thickness

If you're wondering what memory foam mattress thickness would best suit you, 10 to 12 inches is ideal. If you weigh under 250 lbs., a 10-inch mattress will suffice. If you or your partner are over 250 lbs., or if you feel you would appreciate the extra thickness, then go for a 12-inch.

I would stay away from 8-inches or under unless you are a skinny teenager.

Myself, I got the thickest one, because I personally thought it to be a little more comfortable.

3. Motion Transfer Reduction

The "Tempur Material" impressively reduces motion transfer, so your partner's sleep movement won't disturb you. If I get up in the middle of the night to get a drink, a snack, or to use the bathroom, my wife doesn't even know I got up. That's pretty beneficial, especially when she is the one getting up, and it's me that's not waking up!

Price range $1,300-$10,000+.

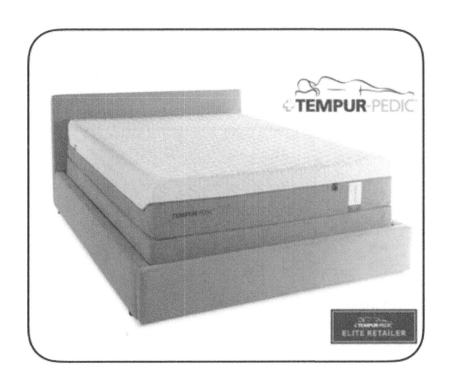

Best mattress for comfort and spinal alignment!

Now, after sleeping on this bed for almost two years, I have had the very best sleeps of my life because it keeps me in….

....**great spinal alignment for eight straight hours!**

Check out these tidbits!

In 1997, MAS (Medical Agency Services) carried out a survey of 2500 physiotherapy patients, that showed that <u>98% of bed purchases were made without any input from a healthcare professional, although they were seeking relief from a medically related condition</u>. (2)

Many <u>European retailers</u> allow purchasers to try a bed or mattress for at least a week. Therefore, in order to rest easier, you may have to insist that the retailer allow you to trial the bed or mattress at home! (3)

In conclusion....

Buying a new bed can be an expensive mistake. It is not just the cost of the bed, but the loss of work, the loss of income to both employer and employee if it causes a disc problem.

Most people will keep a bed for about 10 years. Make sure you don't buy 10 years of avoidable pain! (4)

Dr. G's Tip!

Do you remember the movie *The Graduate* with Dustin Hoffman? At his college graduation party, at poolside, his dad's friend whispered in his ear "plastics". This was to let Dustin know what the next big industry was, to make money in.

So, I am going to whisper, *"medium firm"*. This is the one mattress that I absolutely would test out first! This mattress will support the spine the best, for most people.

Pillow Talk

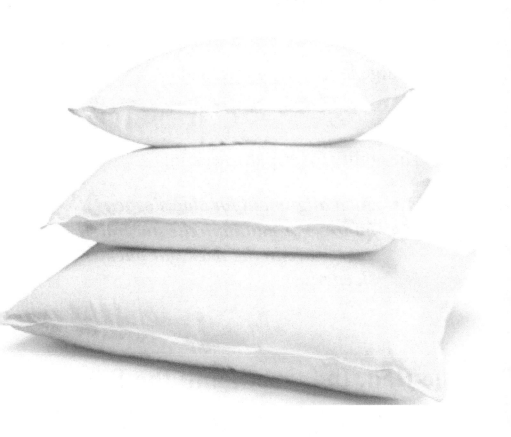

Best Pillows

A good pillow will have these two features:

1. A large level of **_comfort_**, and

2. The ability to keep the neck in:

   - *good alignment for side sleepers*
   - *improve or maintain the natural 45-degree arc in the neck, for back sleepers.*

The Bad, the Good, and the Best!

Now, let's talk about some different pillows. There's a variety that I like and plenty that I have thrown to the curb. Let's start with the bad.

Bad: Feather Pillow

I have used many pillows in my lifetime. I would venture to say at least seven. In my early years, I had a traditional down or feather pillow. Back then, they did not have such a broad range of choices as we do today.

The feather pillow is a basic run-of-the-mill down pillow (below). I would not recommend it, because:

it clearly violates #2, in that it does not improve or maintain the proper arc of the neck.

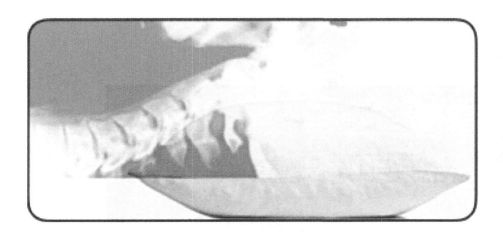

This pillow is too fluffy and may knock your neck right out of alignment!

Good: Egg Crate Pillow

After I graduated from Chiropractic School, I purchased an egg crate pillow. I appreciated how it **maintained the arc** in my neck, and it was definitely better than my down pillow, but for some reason, I still was not jumping up and down about it.

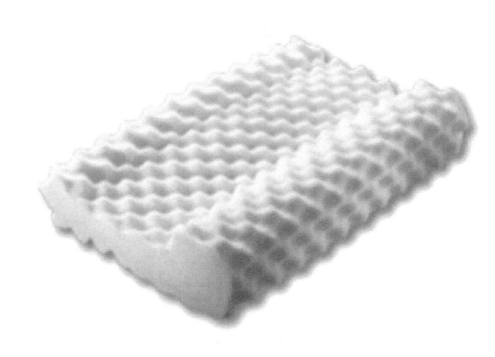

Egg crate pillow is a good pillow.

Better than Good, but still not the Best: Memory Foam Pillow

My next pillow, the memory foam pillow, turned out to be my favorite up to that point. I had some of my best nights of sleep on it. I slept on this pillow for about two years. The only problem that I ran into was, that with time, the foam deflated and smashed down to where it did not support my neck the way it did in the beginning.

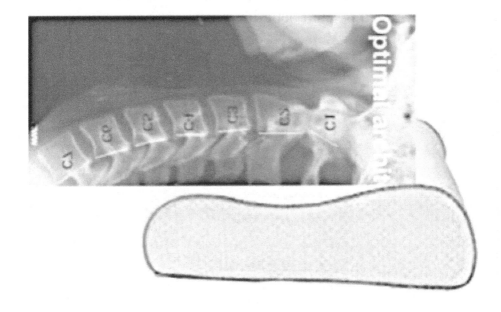

This memory foam pillow improves or maintains the 45-degree cervical arc!

I used this for 2 years.

Best: Tri-Core Pillow

About 20 years ago, a fellow colleague told me about the Tri-core pillow. I bought one and have been using it ever since. The Tri-Core is the pillow I recommend first to my patients. I would estimate that nine out of ten of them liked theirs. That is a pretty good batting average!

My patients liked their Tri-Core so much that many of them bought one for their spouse. So, because of the love I have for this pillow, I wanted to take a little time to talk about the features and benefits.

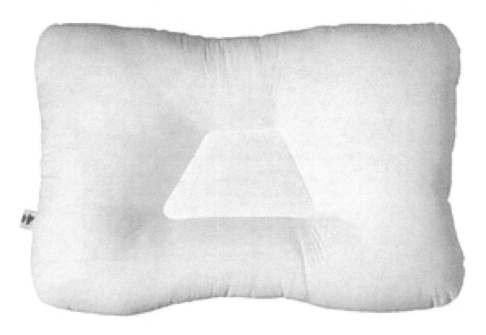

This is a great pillow and is what I sleep on!

Quite a bargain at $50!

Features and Benefits of the Tri-Core

- It is a **fiber pillow** and is **allergy free**. Pillows made from this material generally have a firmer support for your head and neck and tend to last longer than a down or feather pillow.

- The shape of the tri-core pillow **cradles the head and firmly supports the neck**. The benefit of this is that while you are sleeping, your neck will have better alignment, and in some cases may help to restore its natural curve towards 45 degrees.

- If you are a side sleeper, it is **designed to keep your neck in straight alignment**. This is very important, because I would venture to guess that 70% of the population are side sleepers.

- They have **priced this right at around the $50 mark**, which makes it very economical.

Good Tip!

I would purchase it from Amazon rather than directly from Tri-Core, because it costs less, and you get free shipping if you have prime.

I hope this helps in some way and good sleeping!

Take Home Message

✓ A great mattress is one that provides both great support to the spine, while also providing great comfort.

✓ A mattress that is **too soft** will cause the pelvis to sink in the mattress causing increased stresses on the lumbar spine for 6-8 hours a night.

✓ A mattress that is **too firm** will not allow the pelvis and lumbar spine to align properly, causing increased stresses which will eventually lead to back pain and stiffness.

✓ The **best mattress** for most people, in my opinion, is a **medium- firm** mattress. This will allow the pelvis and lumbar spine to stay in good alignment and will result in a good quality sleep every night.

✓ **Best mattress** is the **Tempur-Pedic**.

✓ **Best pillow** is the **Tri-Core** ($50) that can be purchased from Amazon.com

STEP 7

Aligning and Decompressing the Spine: The Final Step

Two roads diverged in a wood, and I-
I took the road less traveled by,
And that has made all the difference.

-Robert Frost

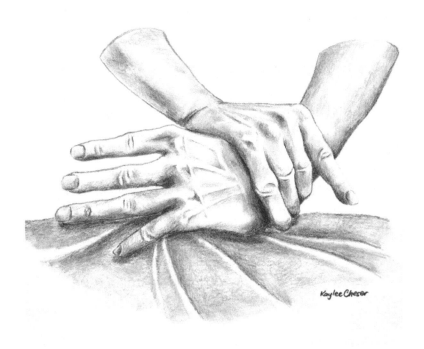

To have a healthy, pain-free back, one final ingredient will be necessary: a de-compressed and aligned spine.

Recently, a patient in his mid 50's entered my clinic complaining of back and leg pain he has had for six years. The last three years though, his pain had intensified, and it was radiating down his right leg to the bottom of his foot. He was currently taking pain pills, so he could continue to work.

His examination revealed a strong core, good arches and posture. He told me he purchased a new bed about three years ago when his back pain started to get worse. He was active and had been exercising most of his life three-to four times a week. He told me he hydrates well, drinking 3/4 gallon of water a day!

Usually when I examine a patient, I usually find some complicating factors such as weight, a weak core, a fallen arch, and or bad posture. In his case though, it was just the opposite. He looked like an absolute picture of health, like that of a competitive tennis player.

His x-rays told the story!

As soon as I looked at his x-rays, though, it was easy to see why he was in pain. His bottom lumbar bones were out of alignment (see next page). It looked like they had been stuck and out of position for twenty plus years because the discs between the same out of aligned bones, had noticeable wear and tear on them (see next page). To have this much wear and tear they had to be compressed and out of alignment a long time.

I saved this story for the last chapter because a healthy pain-free back will usually require one final ingredient: the spine to be de-compressed and in good alignment!

You can easily see his lower spine is compressed and out of alignment.

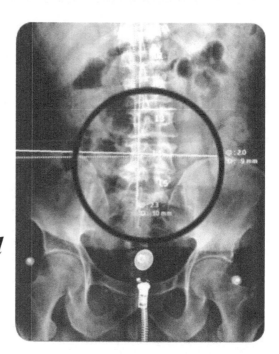

See how his bottom two discs are worn.

This has caused a lack of space for the sciatic nerve and was pinching it.

The sciatic nerve runs down the leg to the foot.

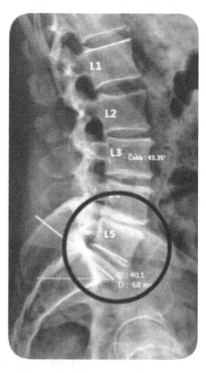

His pain was eliminated in 90 days with spinal adjustments.

What exactly is a chiropractic adjustment?

Chiropractic adjustments are the application of a universal law:

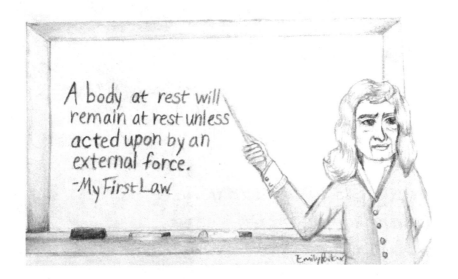

Newton's First Law of Motion: In my profession it could read:

- *Compressed and mis-aligned spinal bones at rest, pinching a nerve,*
- *will remain at rest, continuing to pinch the nerve,*
- *unless it is acted upon by an external force (an adjustment).*

Chiropractors <u>move back into alignment</u>:

- compressed, and

- out of aligned spinal bones, that are
- pinching nerves,

<u>thereby, restoring nerve flow</u> (see pages 182-183).

I do this procedure usually with my hands or an adjusting instrument.

Here I am using my neuromechanical instrument.

It employs 90 lbs. of force, which is the force required to decompress the lumbar spinal bones.

This is very safe and pain-free!

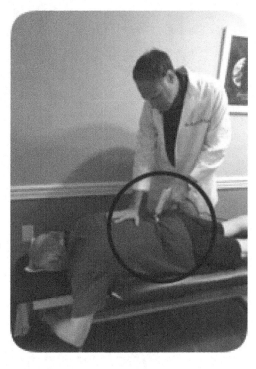

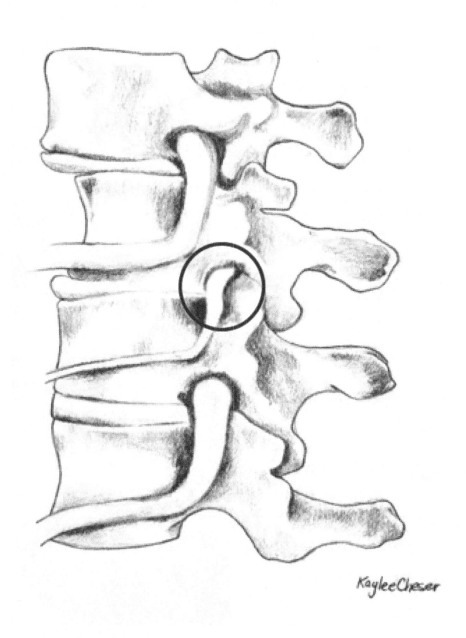

Pinched nerve caused by a
compressed and mis-aligned spine.

Here is what the adjustment does:

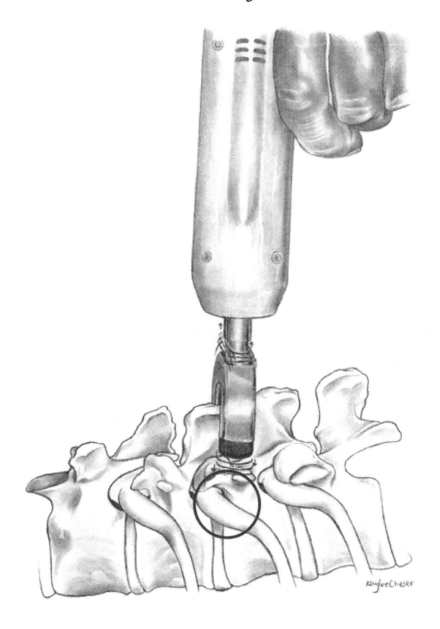

de-compresses and *aligns* the spinal
bones, thereby un-pinching the nerve.

Pills will not move the bone off the nerve!

Pills do not correct pinched nerves, whether they are over the counter or prescriptions, because they will not move the bone or disc away from the pinched nerve. They only can numb the area at best.

Some of these OTC's and prescriptions may mask the problem for a while, especially anti-inflammatories, when the joints and disc have low mileage. However, when the odometer starts to click off the miles, the disc starts to collapse, the jelly material bulges into the nerve, and the joints start to become arthritic from all the stress, then these pills won't get it done!

The usual narrative I hear: "I am taking OTC's, prescriptions, shots and I still hurt!"

Most people that have back pain do not call me first. The typical story I am told is they tried the Ibuprofen and heating pad first. They do this for a few weeks. Then they go to their local doctor and they get a prescription. If that does not get rid of their pain, the doctor may refer them for a few rounds of physical therapy. If that does not do it, they usually get an MRI, get referred to pain management and get steroid injections. If they still aren't getting better, they may consult with a neurosurgeon or may even call a chiropractor.

So, by the time they come to my office, they have been everywhere else without any help. They often arrive with an MRI report in their hands, that has **"disc desiccation"**, **"degeneration"**, **"bulges"**, **"stenosis"**, **"bone spurring"**, **"facet hypertrophy"**, **"osteophyte formations"**, **"foraminal narrowing"**, written all over it!

200

Typical MRI Report. The patient needs a Latin translator for this stuff!!!

Spinal adjustments: the procedure that should be done before medicine, shots and surgery.

The only wise thing left to do, after taking all the drugs and doing the shots, is what should have been done in the first place:

- re-align the spine,
- decompress and re-hydrate the disc, and
- remove the nerve pressure.

And then hope for the best, because the doctor waiting at the very end of the line is the neurosurgeon, who has a handful of screws!

A word about maintaining spinal care.

When a patient's back gets better from spinal adjusting, it is not uncommon for them to ask, "Dr. Graham, do I have to have my spine adjusted forever?"

My answer is always, "of course you don't".

However, outlined below are few things to think about, before you decide on whether or not you want to maintain the alignment of your spine:

- ✓ If you once had chronic back pain you are more likely than someone who has never had it, to go under the knife.

- ✓ Cost: A lumbar fusion surgery combined with medications, MRI, rehabilitation, and time off work approaches $170,000. (1)

- ✓ Off work: With fusion surgeries, the patient will usually be off work four to six weeks to rest their back. (2)

- ✓ Rehabilitation time: Time consuming and costly.

- ✓ Full recovery time: 3-6 months, depending on your age, overall health and physical condition. (2)

- ✓ Success rate: If you define "success" as some reduction of pain, then 30%-40% are not successful. (3)

- ✓ Complications: These include infection, bleeding, anesthetic complications and nerve damage. (3)

202

Case Studies

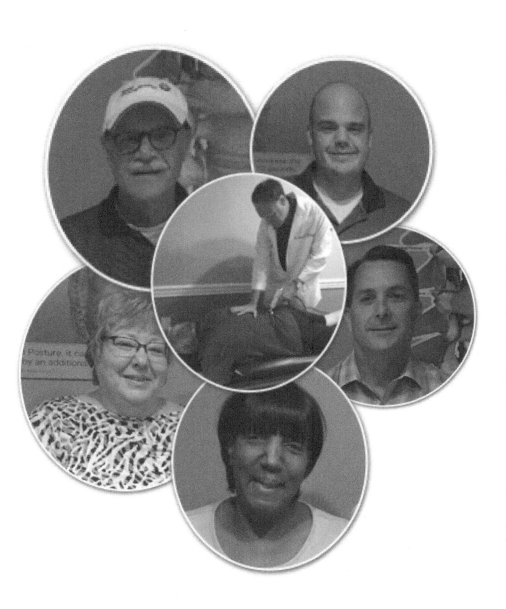

Case study #1

This is the story of Sam.

Highlights of case

Chief complaint: _LOWER BACK Sholder_

Date it started _1 / 12/16_ Cause _In SURE Yers of Concrete work_

if injury, where did it happen:_____

Pain Diagram

Please mark the area of injury or discomfort on the chart below:

ease use the space below to describe your condition further if needed:

When dewing Sharp Pain Around hip down the Left Leg

- **Problem**: back and leg pain for 2 years.

- **Pills**: Meloxicam and Advil

- **Other**: heating pad, ice pack, sits on a pillow when he drives

- **Worse with**: sitting, driving, walking, bending, laying on his back

- Head on collision 40+ years ago and works on concrete.

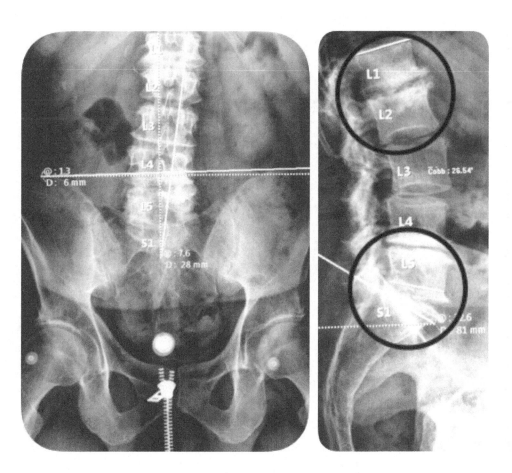

X-rays showed: See above

- A high left hip
- A moderate misalignment at L4-5
- Worn out discs in his lower back (L1-2; L4-5; L5-S1)

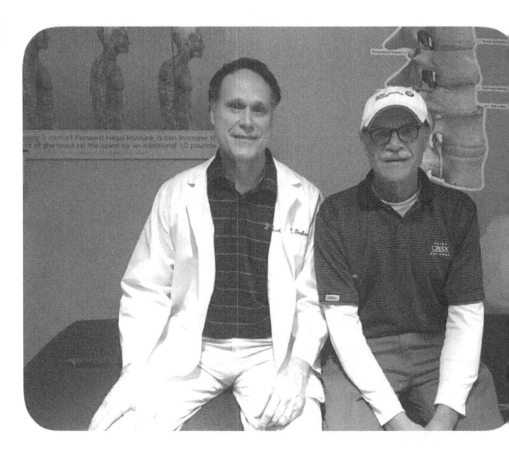

Sam and me

Sam's leg pain was totally gone after one month!

He is maintaining his spine and disc once a month.

Case study #2

This is the story of Tracey.

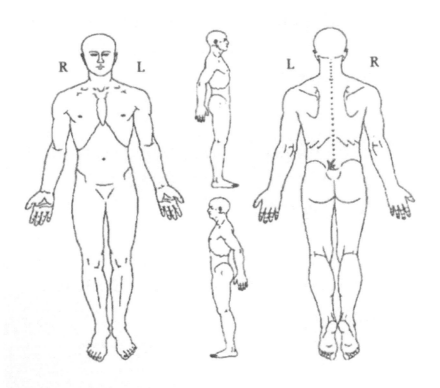

Please use the space below to describe your condition further if needed: _____

SHARP PAIN ON OCCASION, SEVERE PAIN SHOOTING DOWN
MY LEFT LEG

Highlights of case

- **Problem**: back pain and severe sharp shooting pain in his left buttock and thigh almost every time he stood up from the seated position

- **Tried**: Ibuprofen; putting a pillow in the small of his back; stretching; and exercising (planks)

- **Worse with**: standing up from the seated position

- **X-rays**: showed two discs that were collapsing (L4-5 and L5-S1)

This side view shows that he has almost totally worn out his disc at L4-5

Probably took 30 years to wear out that much!

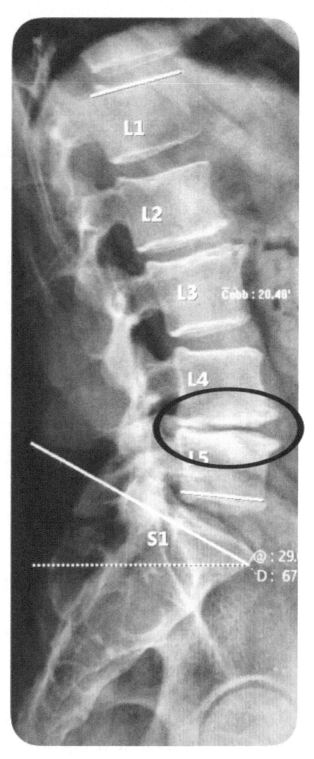

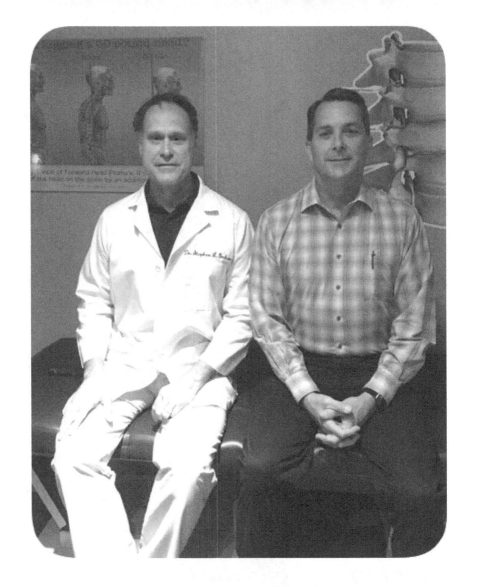

Tracey and me

After 45 days his pain in his leg was totally gone!

He keeps his spine de-compressed twice a month, so his disc does not collapse anymore.

Case study #3

This is the story of William.

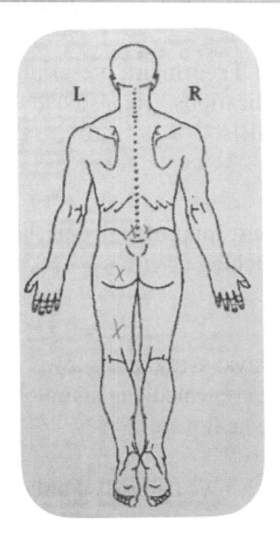

Highlights of case

- **Problem**: For the last 5 years his back and leg have hurt, but this time it was so severe that he had to start curtailing activities, including golf!

- **Past Treatment**: prescription medications. He also had undergone 2 MRIs.

- **Tried**: Ibuprofen, ice packs, and stretching

- **X-rays**: x-ray of his lower lumbar discs revealed degeneration at L4-5 (see next page).

- **MRI**: revealed a disc bulge at L4-5.

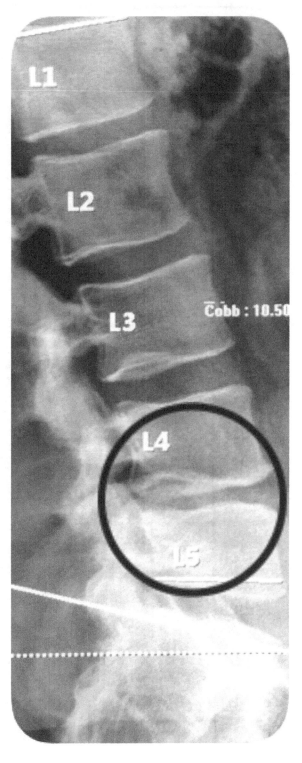

Disc Degeneration.

He is only 26 years old!

215

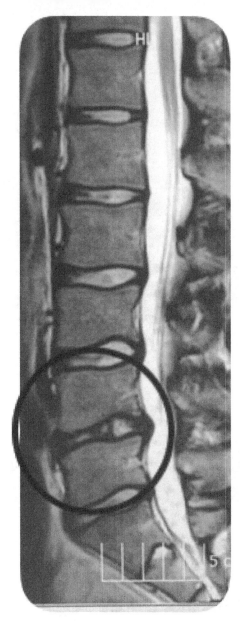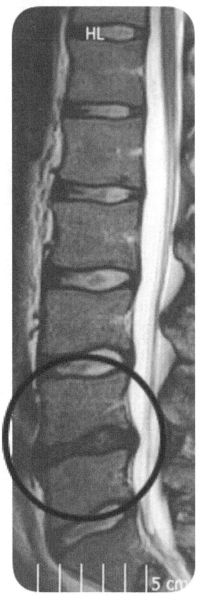

MRI from 2013 and 2015.

Notice how much darker the L4-5 disc has gotten in just two years (dehydrating)!

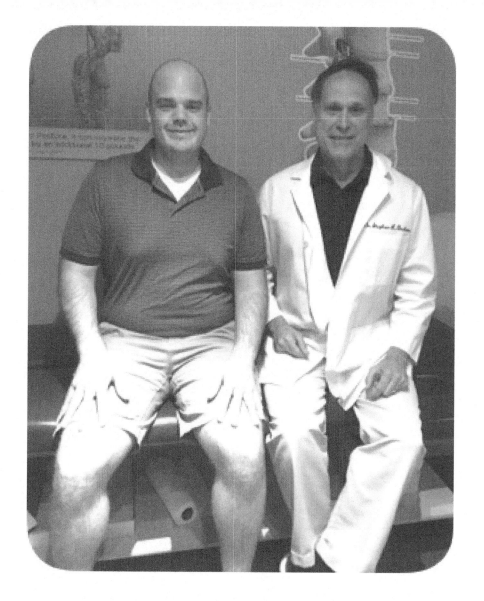

Will and me

For the first time in 5 long years, Will's leg pain is gone, and he is golfing again!!!

He keeps his spine de-compressed and aligned once a month to prevent further degeneration.

Case study #4

This is the story of Karen.

This case was very interesting because I believe it was an example of both a bad disc and a fallen arch that contributed to her back and leg pain.

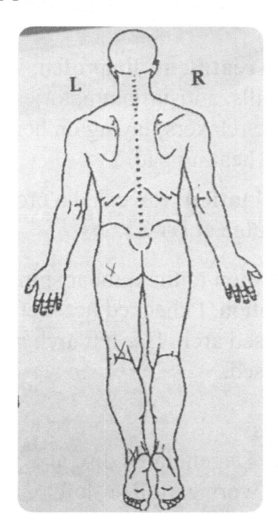

Highlights of case

- **Problem**: Back and left leg pain that radiated all the way to her ankle. This has been present on and off, for 2-3 years. It got worse at the end of January (01-25-18) when she woke.

- **Past Treatment**: Ibuprofen; Tylenol, pain pills, anti-inflammatories, muscle relaxers; laying on her back used a heating pad.

- **Examination**: Revealed a probable disc bulge at L5-S1.

  In addition to the lumbar spine evaluation, I checked her feet for a collapsed arch. Her left arch was collapsed.

- **X-rays**:
  Spine: Degenerated disc at L5-S1
  Knee: worn cartilage -left

You can see how the very bottom disc has lost much of its tread.

This is similar to what happens to a tire on a car when it is out of alignment!

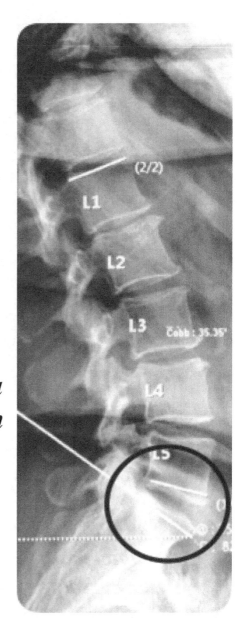

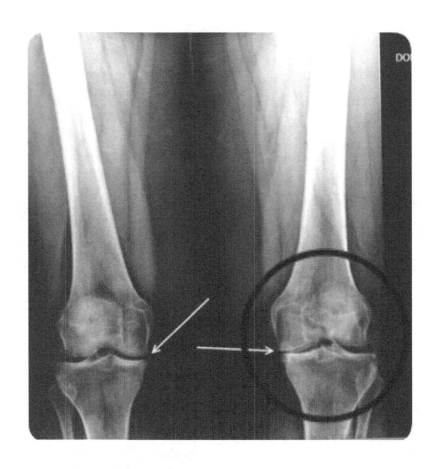

Notice the worn-out cartilage on the inside of the left knee (circled)!

She had been told she needed a knee replacement, but she did not want to put herself at risk with surgery.

I prescribed orthotics.
Shortly thereafter, her knee pain left!

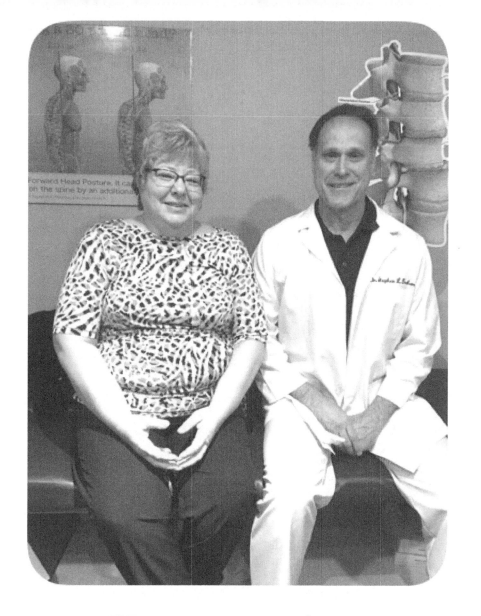

Karen and me

She is smiling because she can walk up and down her steps without any pain in her back, leg or knee!!

Case study #5

This is the story of Kelley.

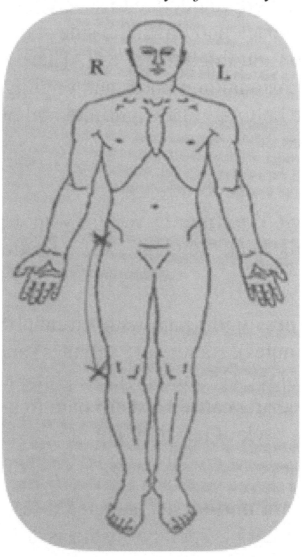

Chief complaint: _____
Date it started 12 / 1 / 16 Cause Repetitive motion
If injury, where did it happen: Driving my bus (Substitute
School bus)

All past surgeries:

<u>Highlights of case</u>

- **Problem**: moderate to severe pain in her low back and down the side and back of her right thigh to her calf. There was occasional numbness and tingling into the bottom of her right foot and outer toes.

- **Past Treatment**: Advil, Tylenol, pain pills, heat, "Icy Hot", and a heating pad

- **Worse with:** pain with sitting (10 minutes), standing (5 minutes) and walking (15 minutes); coughing and sneezing caused a sharp pain to go down the back of her right leg

- **Examination**: degenerated discs at L4-5 and L5-S1; spondylolisthesis at L4 on L5 Grade I

Two worn out discs at:

- *L4-L5 and*
- *L5-S1*

L4 has slipped forward.

This slippage stretches the nerve!

See drawings on next page.

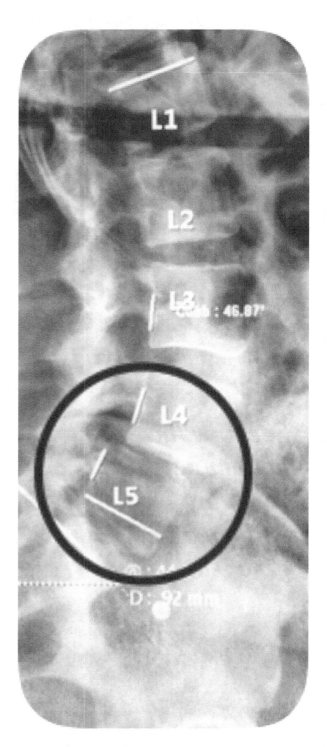

Spondylolisthesis=Slip

See how the bone has slipped forward!

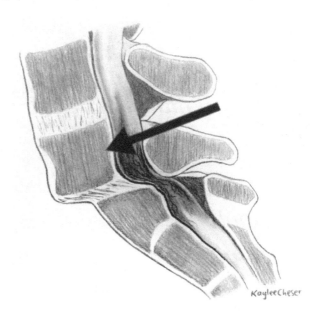

See how the bottom nerve is getting stretched and pinched!

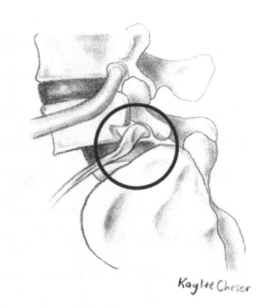

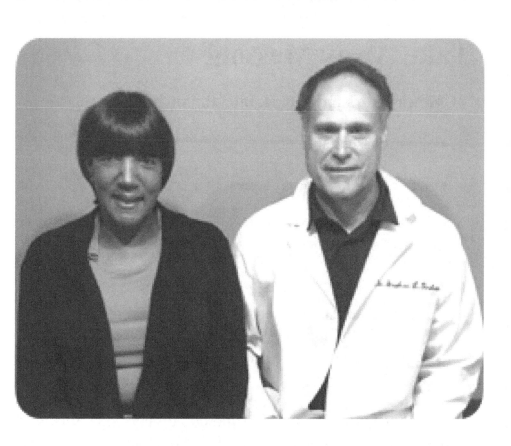

Kelley and me

Kelley is happy that she is able to drive her bus pain-free!!!

She maintains the health of her two bad discs by getting adjustments two times a month.

Take Away Message

✓ **Chiropractors <u>move back into alignment</u>**:

- compressed, and

- out of aligned spinal bones, that are
- pinching nerves,

<u>**thereby, restoring nerve flow**</u> **(see pages 182-183).**

✓ **Periodic spinal adjustments** serve as a preventative measure to help increase the chances of **preventing future back pain.**

✓ **Spinal adjustments are safe** and do not have side effects such as liver or kidney damage that can occur with even OTC drugs.

✓ **Prevention**! Just like Dr. Weber stated in the foreword to this book, the best way to have a strong, healthy pain-free back is prevention. The odds are strongly against you, if you do nothing.

In conclusion

Today, I am writing this book totally pain-free. I know what it is like to be in pain as I lived with back and leg pain for 28 months. The worst thing about it was that I was sidelined from sports! When my friends were playing basketball, tennis and golf, I was miserable not being able to participate. I have never forgotten that feeling.

So, in 1983, after my very first spinal adjustment, I knew I was going to have my spine aligned and balanced for the rest of my life. Here are just a few of the ways adjustments have benefitted me over the past 35 years!

✓ *Kept my spine in alignment.*

✓ *Re-hydrated my discs to prevent premature degeneration, disc bulging and any other damage.*

✓ *Helped to keep my posture erect.*

✓ *Improved my balance and strength.*

✓ *Helped me sustain a drug-free life.*

✓ *Kept me active and pain-free!*

The following pages show just a few of the activities I can enjoy because I have invested the time to take care of my spine!

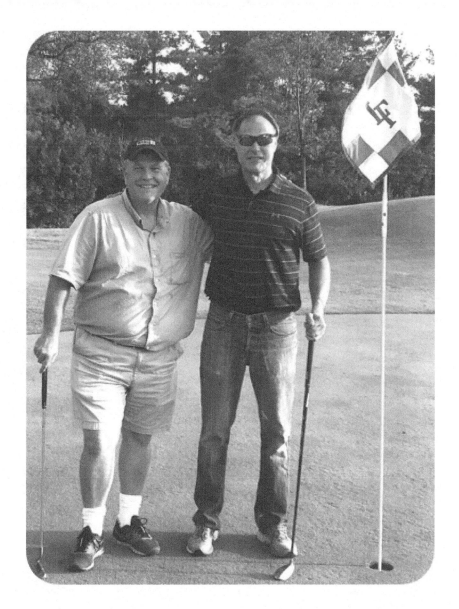

My great friend Mark Cowherd and me playing double bogey to triple bogey golf!

Golf really tests the spine with the bending and torquing!

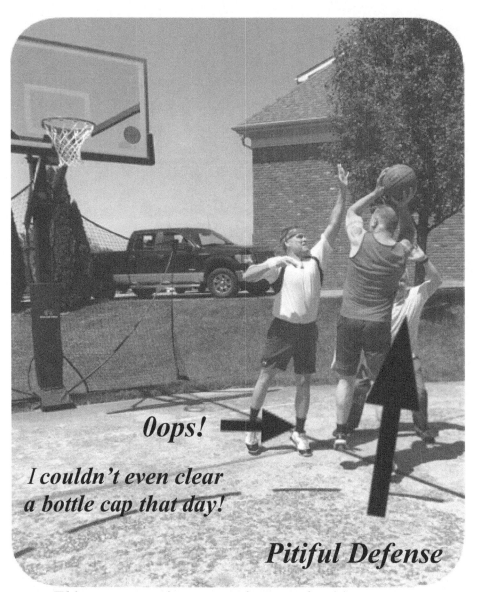

Oops!

*I couldn't even clear
a bottle cap that day!*

Pitiful Defense

This sport requires a good strong back!

*Bernie Lubbers (shooter), Owen Caster (guy that is
playing pitiful defense), and me (barely jumping
off the ground), playing "21" in my backyard.*

I think that awkward shot actually went in!

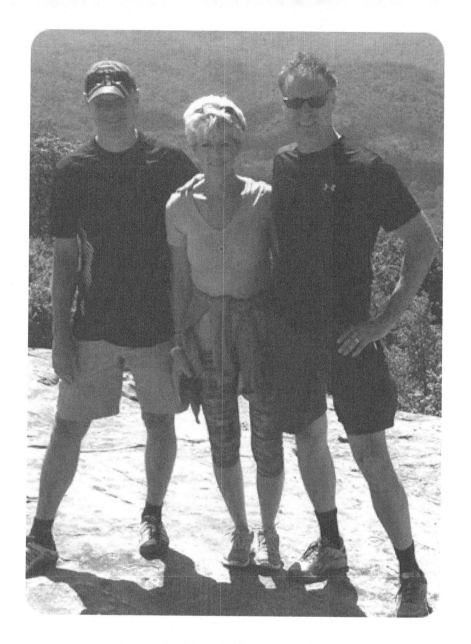

Hiking requires a good strong core!

Here we are in the tall mountains of North Carolina!

The good-looking blonde is my wife, Donna.

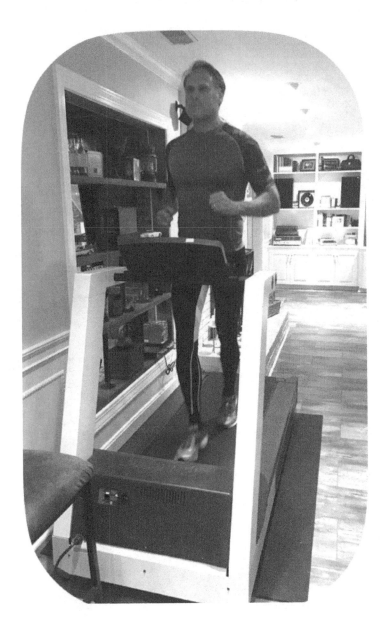

Let's face it, if your spine is wearing out, you probably have to give up sprinting!

No disrespect to Edison, but I think the treadmill is the greatest invention of them all!

No, he is not spoiled!

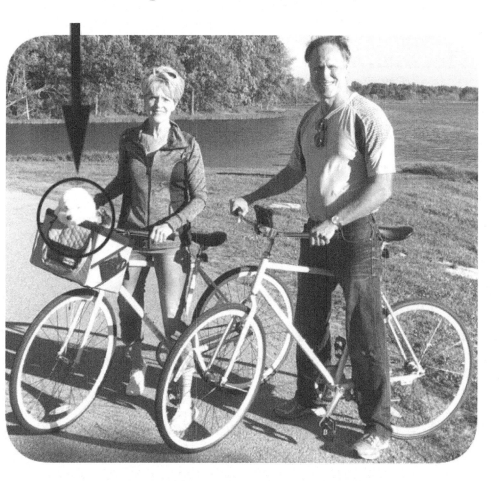

You have to have a top-notch spine to ride bikes, especially when you are hauling the little guy along!

One Final Note:

According to the American Chiropractic Association, only 10% of the population use a chiropractor!

My Open Letter to the 10 Percenters!

Dear 10%er's,

Thank you for taking the path less traveled; for being courageous in the face of your friends or family, who may have laughed at you for thinking different!

You are definitely the round pegs in the square holes! You are the fearless ones! You are the heroes who will leave a family legacy, that says no to DRUGS!

Congratulations on being the crazy 10%'ers!

Stephen h. Graham
— D.C. —

TOP 10
"Jacked-Up"
Spines of the Year!

After growing up watching David Letterman's TOP 10, I thought it might be fun to research the "TOP 10 Jacked-Up Spines of the Year!" I thought this would be a neat way to show some really messed up spines that most people would never get a chance to see. In addition, it may make you feel a little better knowing that at least 10 people have a more jacked-up spine than you have!

Once I decided on this task, I spent what seemed like, at least two days exhaustively reviewing all the x-rays from 2017. This turned out to be quite the job. My first cut included 75 x-rays. I then narrowed it down to 30. Then it got tough.

I put the project aside for a few days and then came back to it. I then narrowed it down to the top 20. After this, my eyes were just not working right, so I asked my wife what she thought. When I first asked her for help, she said, "Are you still fooling around with that jacked-up spine thing"! In spite of her cute comment, she helped me anyway and together, we got my top 10!

Then I had to put it in order, from best to worst, which took me another few hours. So, after getting them all in order, naturally, I started questioning myself and I thought, "Steve, just go with it!"

So, here they are: The 10 most "Jacked-Up" Spines of the Year!"

"Honorable Mention"

Two giant bulges causing back and leg pain for 9 years!

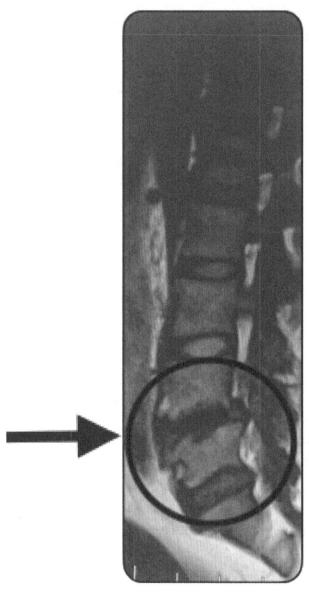

- White discs are hydrated and healthy!

- These black discs are weaker and can bulge, herniate and collapse!

- See the two-disc bulges.

- That is why it is important to keep the discs hydrated with spinal adjustments!

#10
16-year old makes the list!

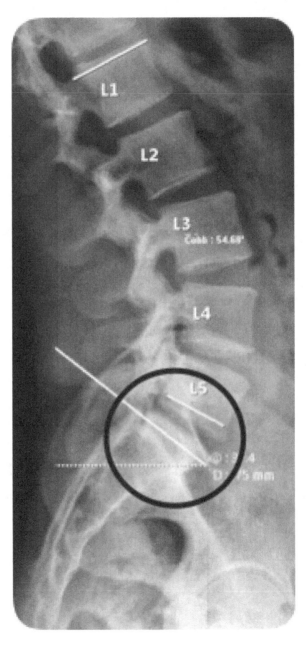

Normally, this would be just an average case. What made it so unusual, was that this nice young man, was just a sophomore in high school!

- He has had back and left leg pain that radiated to his foot since he was 12 years old! He cannot sit or stand more than 10 minutes!

- He was taking pain pills; an anti-inflammatory; and a muscle relaxer.

- My x-ray showed arthritic change at the L4-5, and degeneration at L5-S1.

- The MRI also confirms degenerative disc disease!

1. Left facet arthropathy and left paracentral and foraminal disc protrusion at L4-L5 cause moderate left neural foraminal narrowing and narrowing of the left latera...
2. ...d degenerative disc disease at L5-S1 with out significant spinal canal or neu... ...minal narrowing.

Now, that is Jacked-Up!!!

#9

Broke her bone falling off a horse!

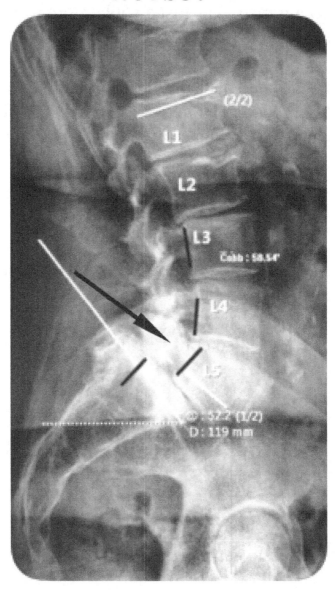

- She has had on and off pain for 50+ years.

- She said it hurt ever since she fell off a horse at age 12.

- You will notice L5 has slipped forward on her sacrum.

   -Lines should be over each other!

   -This is referred to as a Grade II spondylolisthesis (slipped bone).

- This usually occurs when the bone is broken.

- Often times it will take a hard force to break a bone like falling off a horse, as she did when she was 12.

- Weight gain can pull the slipped bone more forward.

#8
Rusted out spine!

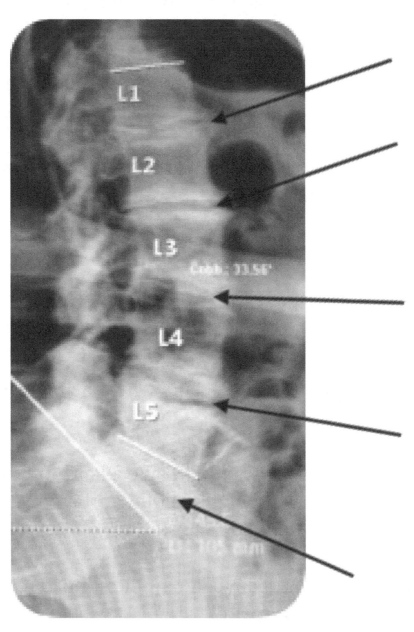

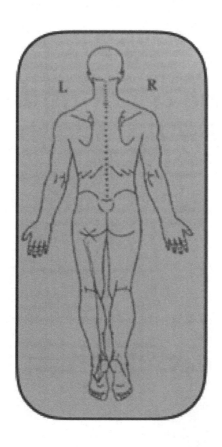

- 4 months of severe back and leg pain.

- This woman's entire lumbar spine is bone on bone.

- Spinal stenosis is a common outcome.

- People that have this generally have a difficult time walking any distances.

#7
Her bone is falling halfway off her spine!

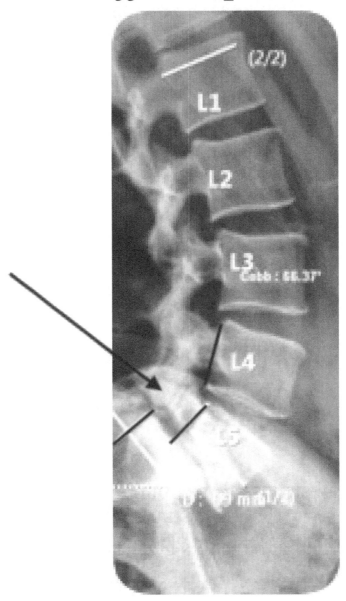

- See how the lines are not on top of each other.

  Bone five has moved forward from S1.

  This is a Grade II spondylolisthesis.

  That means the bone slipped 26-50% off the spine! I see maybe only 3-4 of these a year.

- Normally, it takes a fracture from a hard fall for the bone to begin to slip forward on the spine.

- Most often it takes at least 20 years for the disc to collapse.

- Her bottom disc has <u>collapsed</u> from all the stress and she is only 45 years old!

#6

Look at that big 'ole honkin disc bulge!!!

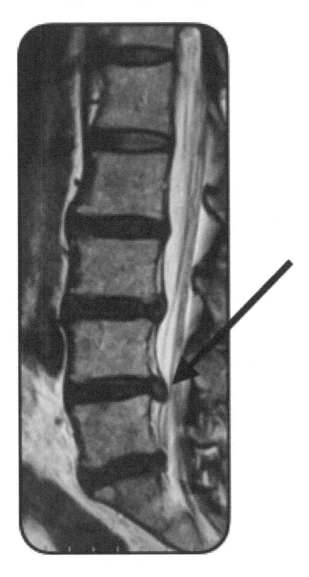

- Severe back pain for months on months!

- Did the following:
  ✓ Ibuprofen
  ✓ muscle relaxers;
  ✓ three epidural shots;
  ✓ compression belt.

- I have read in my scientific journals that a 7mm protrusion is a cut off point for surgery (rule of thumb).

- This one is 6mm. Notice all the black discs!

- Regular x-rays will not show the inside of the disc.

- MRI is the test that gets this done. Bring your wallet! $1,500!

#5

Whoa! Two slipped bones with a collapsed disc!

(1)

(2)

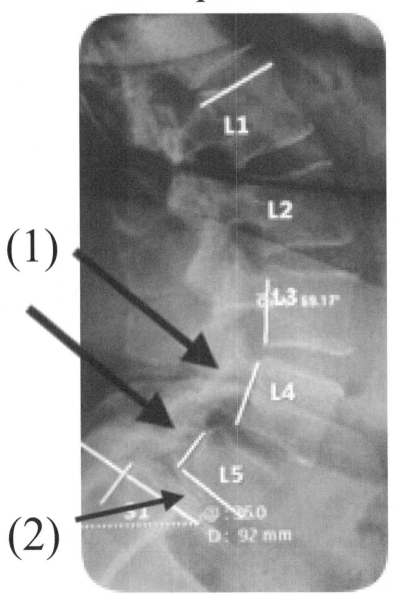

- Fell 20 years ago and fractured her lower back.

- Has had on and off back issues ever since.

- Her pain is going down her L hip and leg.

- (1) See how the bones are sliding forward (double offset).

- This stresses out the bone and disc causing **(2)** disc collapse, bulges and herniations.

- Spondylolisthesis-Grade I and II

#4

Bone on bone at age 47 and has no clue why!

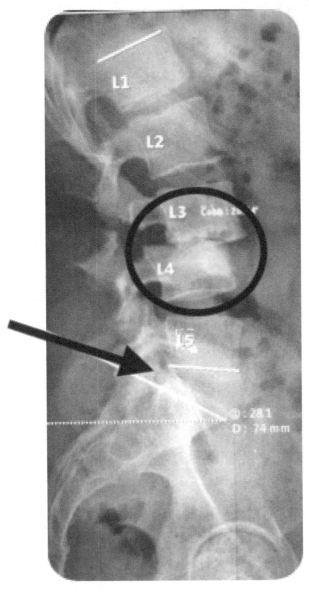

- He has had pain since 2011.

- He has been taking Ibuprofen (8 per day) for at least a year!
  He is one lucky guy that he has not had a bleeding stomach ulcer yet.

- He completely wore out the disc between lumbar bone 3 and 4, probably from bone 3 slipping forward **(circle)**.

- Interestingly, exam findings revealed a pinched nerve at L5-S1,
  not at the "bone on bone" area **(arrow)**.

#3

Largest herniation I have ever seen on MRI, but the pain is from 3 discs below!

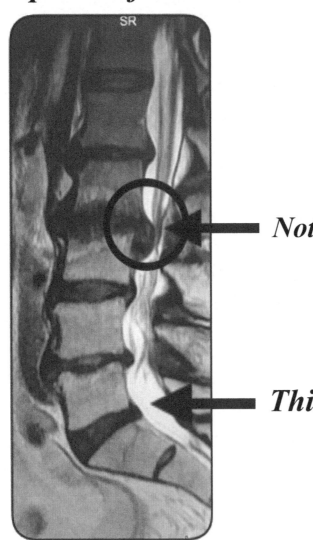

Not this one!

This one!

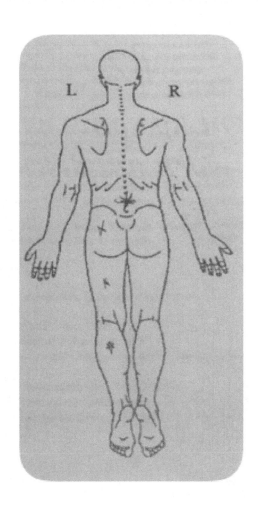

This is why you treat the person,
not the MRI.

#2
Bent up spine with 5 worn out discs!

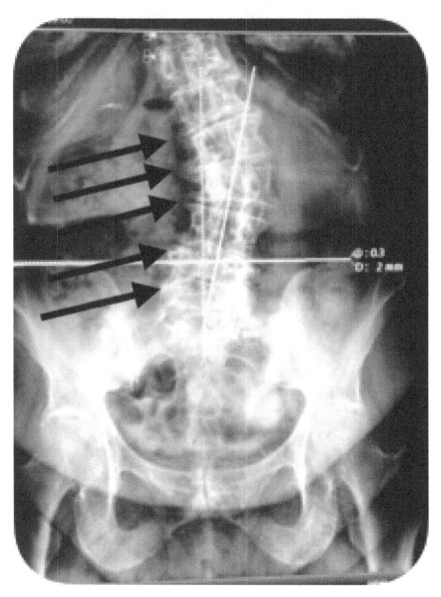

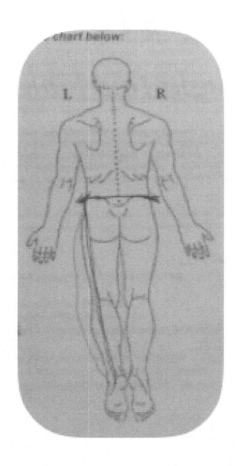

- 25 years of on and off pain!

- Can only sit for 5 minutes; walk for 2 minutes

- Five worn out discs!

- Living on Aleve.

#1
I thought this took it!

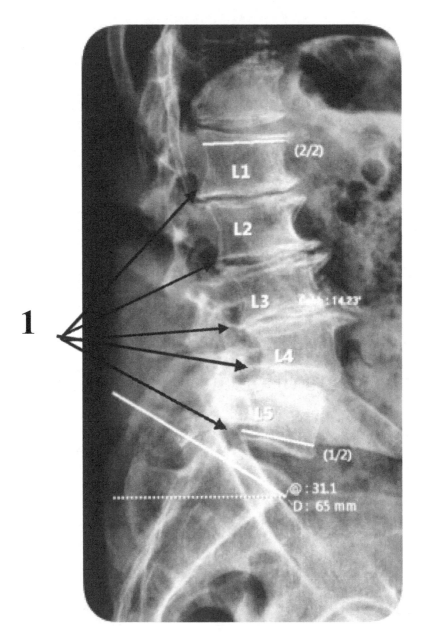

1

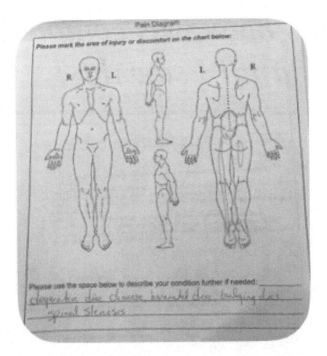

- This man has had on and off pain for 20 years. He injured his back approximately 20 years ago when he fell 7 feet off scaffolding.

- His spine is severely misaligned.

- L4 has slipped forward on L5 (spondylolisthesis).

- His surgeon was talking about rods and screws.

- He also has **(1)** multiple degenerated and bulging discs with spinal stenosis.

This book was complete until I saw this!

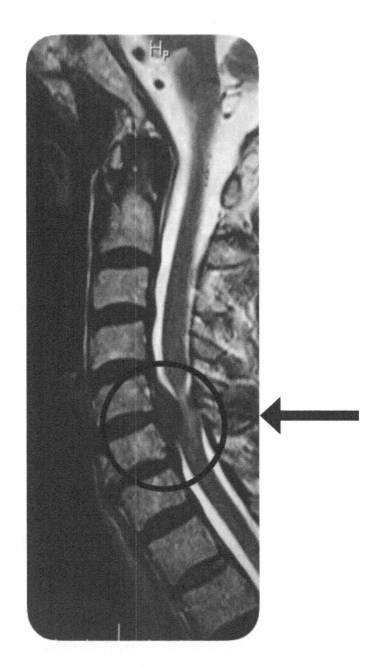

This nice lady came in my office complaining of both neck and back pain. She brought a copy of her MRI from 2011 and I could not believe what I saw! It was the biggest herniation I have ever seen!

She said at the time this was taken in 2011, she was having pain in her right arm and leg.

It is unusual to have pain in both the upper and lower extremities from one cause. When this does happen, more times than not, the problem originates in the cervical spine (neck).

Her chiropractor at that time ordered an MRI of her neck. That same day she went in for an emergency surgery!

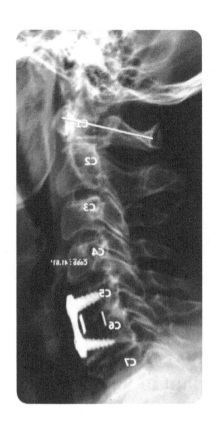

She said her surgeon told her that he had never seen so much pressure on the spinal cord without the person being paralyzed!

In this case, her fusion surgery may have saved her life!

And, that is why this is my new

#1!

BONUS MATERIAL II

HOLY TITANIUM!

Congratulations, you are almost done with *"Don't Get the Screws Put to You!"* I thought it would be fitting at this point to show you some of my patients that literally had the screws put to them.

I made sure to include a few different types of fusions, along with a few relevant facts about each case. I was as shocked as you probably will be, when you see some of these surgeries. I find it interesting, that I am still affected the same way today, as I was in 1988, when I first laid my eyes on a spinal fusion!

Hopefully, this chapter and handbook will help guide you through your decision-making process. Please share this chapter with someone that you know who may be facing back surgery. Hopefully it will make them think twice about getting back surgery or it will motivate them to get a second, third or yet even fourth opinion!

So, I hope you enjoy this last chapter, *Holy Titanium!* as much as I did writing it!

3 back surgeries!

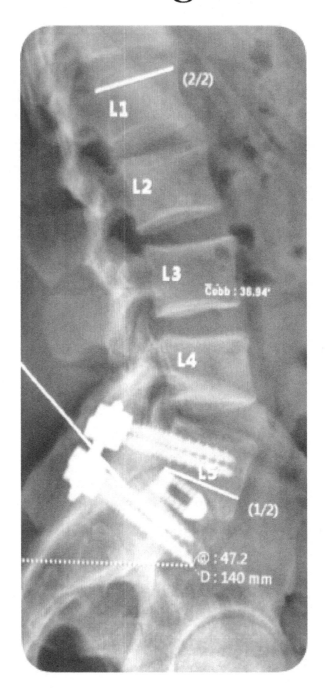

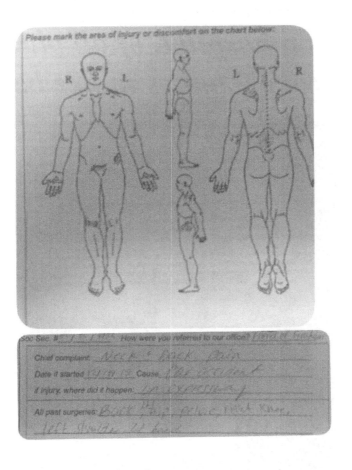

The cost of a single-level spinal fusion surgery depends on a few factors such as the state in which the surgery is performed, the severity of the injury, and the recovery time spent in the hospital. *Spine-health* gives a general range of $90,000 to $160,000 (the cost of a house), as of 2015.

Typical recovery time following the surgery is three to six months, according to *The Rothman Institute*.

Fell at a hospital, of all places, and broke 2 bones in her back!

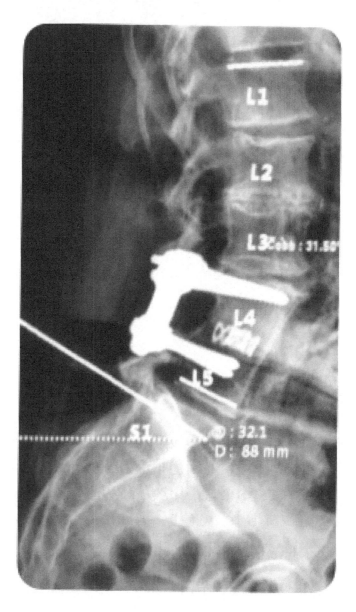

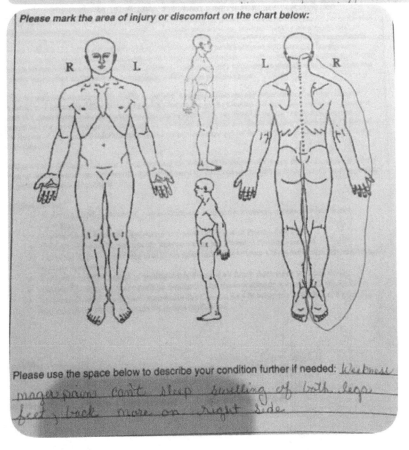

Chief complaint: 4+5 Lumbar surgy meddd platts lots of pain weekness in legs + back
Date it started 11/04/96 Cause Crush spien

Please mark the area of injury or discomfort on the chart below:

Please use the space below to describe your condition further if needed: Weekness major pain, can't sleep swelling of both legs, feet, back more on right side.

Having pain and weakness in her back ever since her fall in 1996.

Taking 5 Ibuprofens a day, wearing a back brace, and rubbing on Bio-Freeze.

16 Advil a day, and that is after the surgery!

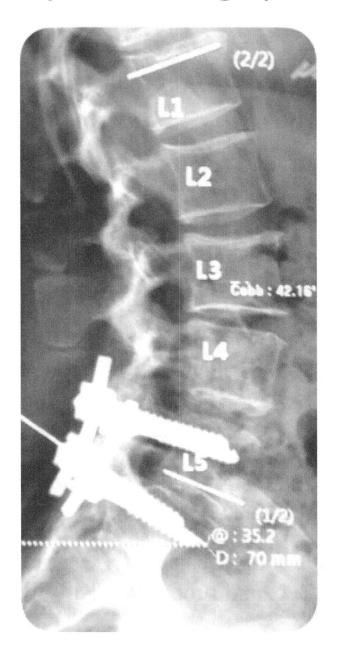

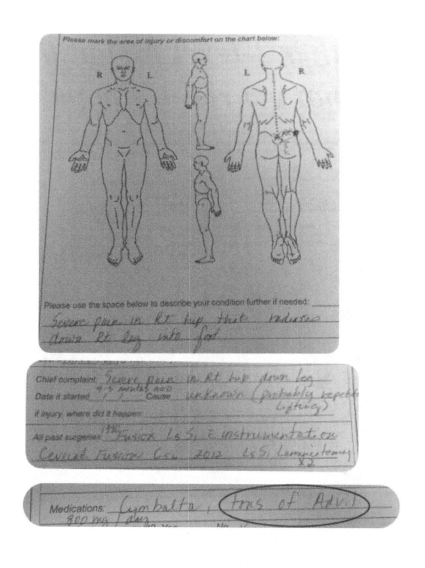

Please mark the area of injury or discomfort on the chart below:

Please use the space below to describe your condition further if needed: _____

Severe pain in Rt hip that radiates down Rt leg into foot

Chief complaint: Severe pain in Rt hip down leg
Date it started 4-5 months ago   Cause: unknown (probably repeated lifting)
If injury, where did it happen: _____

All past surgeries: 1990 Fusion L4-5 & instrumentation Cervical Fusion C5-6 2012 L4-5 Laminectomy

Medications: Cymbalta, tons of Advil 800 mg / day

This poor lady had two laminectomy surgeries. The first one occurred in 1990, the second in 1994.

She was taking "tons" of Advil, which equated to 16 a day. That is <u>16 pills</u>, my friend!

Lucky for her, she did not have a bleeding stomach ulcer!

Another 2-level fusion that did not get rid of the pain!

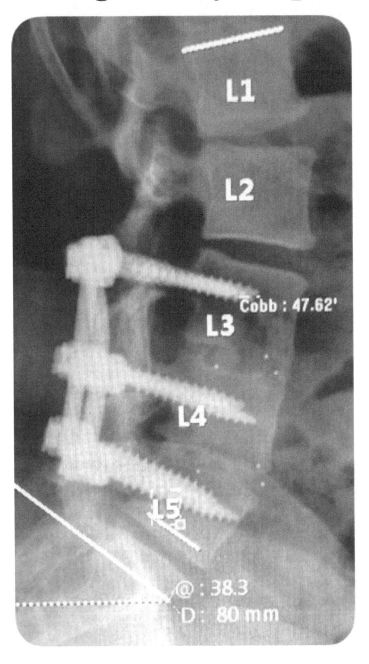

This nice 48-year-old lady worked at the supermarket down the street from my office. When I stopped there to get my morning power bars, she would often times complain about her back pain and how hard it was to stand at the register all day.

I told her to stop in, sometime so I could give it a look.

This is her two-level fusion surgery.

Many times, the level above the surgery starts wearing out. There is no visible degeneration at this point.

She said even after her surgery, some 8 years ago, she still suffers with daily pain!

What's with the key?

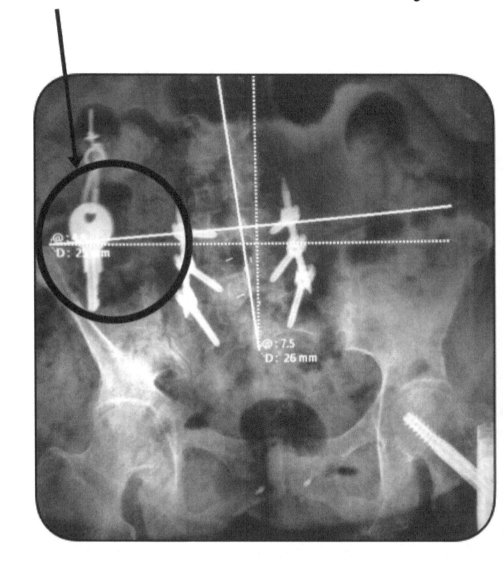

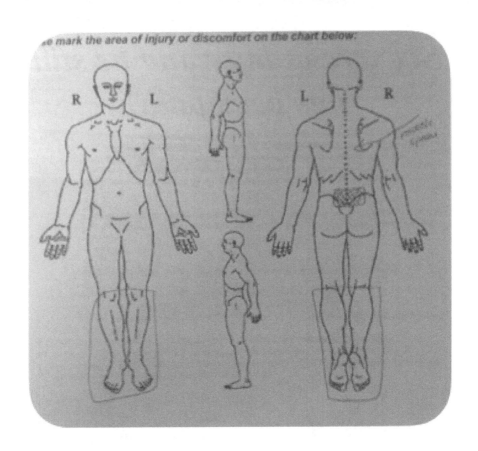

She told me she can only walk or stand for a minute and bending "kills" her back.

She is taking 4 Hydrocodone pills each day!

And by the way, the key should have been removed from her pocket before we took the X-ray. I blamed the assistant, she blamed the patient. Sounds a lot like the home I grew up in!

Six screws later and he still has back pain!

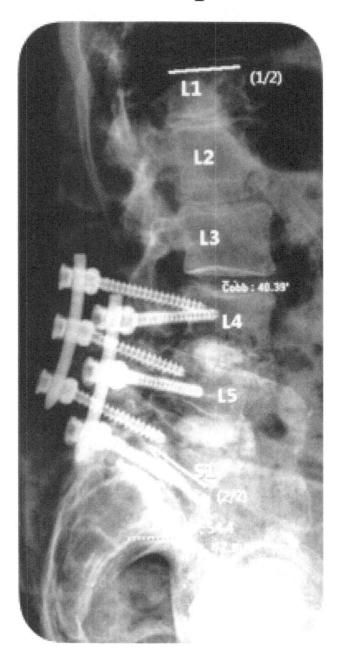

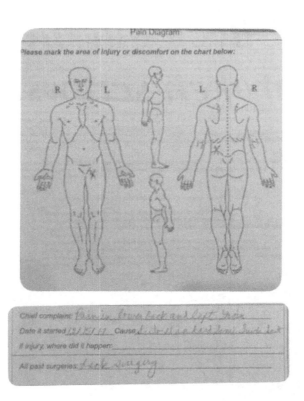

Pain has been present in his low back and groin for the last 4 years. He had surgery 5 years prior. He discussed with me that he has been sitting on "substandard seats" in a semi and thinks that may have caused all this.

For relief he is taking: a steroid pack, 6 Aleve a day, and using a heating pad.

Lumbar fusions of three or more levels of the lower back as a primary treatment for low back pain is rarely recommended. Many surgeons will not perform any more than a single level fusion.

Check out the broken screws!

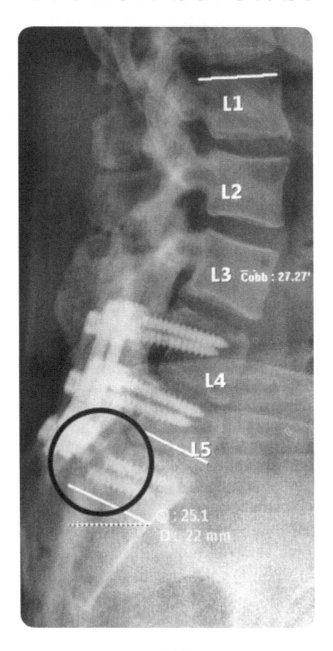

A daughter that had brought her mom in to be treated, asked me if I could look at her back.

She said that she had 5 surgeries to her lower back, over the last 12 years, the last one being a lumbar fusion surgery. A few years ago, she found out that some of the screws had broken.

I took an x-ray of the side of her spine and Lo and Behold, the bottom two screws were broken!

She said the surgeon is afraid to attempt to remove the screws fear of it getting worse than it already is.

Nightmare at the airport security check!

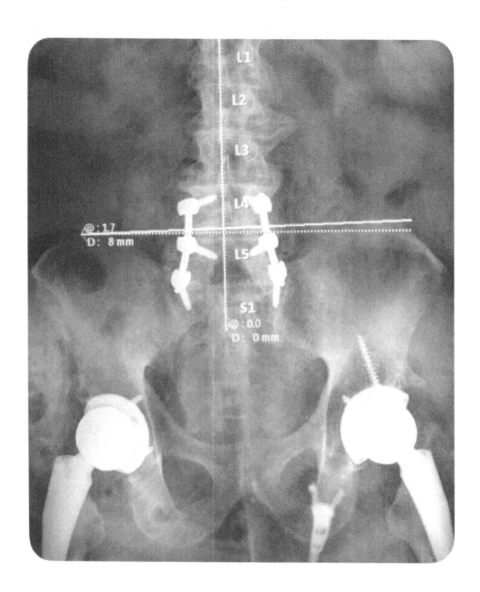

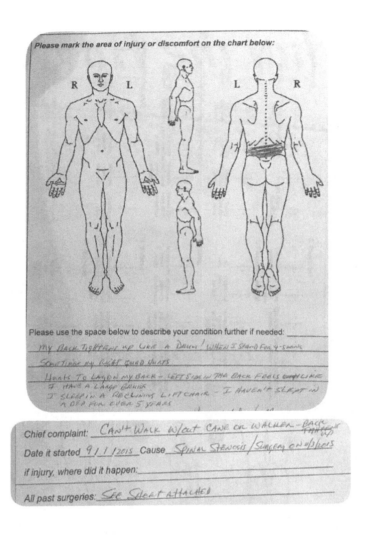

Please mark the area of injury or discomfort on the chart below:

Please use the space below to describe your condition further if needed: _____
MY BACK TIGHTENS UP LIKE A DRUM / WHEN I STAND FOR 4-5 MINS
SOMETIMES MY LEFT QUAD HURTS
Hurts TO LAY ON MY BACK - LEFT SIDE IN THE BACK FEELS EMPTY LIKE
I HAVE A LARGE BRUISE
I SLEEP IN A RECLINING LIFT CHAIR - I HAVEN'T SLEPT IN
A BED FOR OVER 5 YEARS

Chief complaint: CAN'T WALK W/OUT CANE OR WALKER - BACK TIGHTENS (UP)
Date it started 9 / 1 / 2015 Cause SPINAL STENOSIS / SURGERY ON 4/3/2015
if injury, where did it happen: _____

All past surgeries: SEE SHEET ATTACHED

He can only stand five minutes and has instant pain when he walks. It hurts him to lay down, bend forward, twist to either side, or lift.

He has been sleeping in a recliner for 5 years.

What the Hay!!!

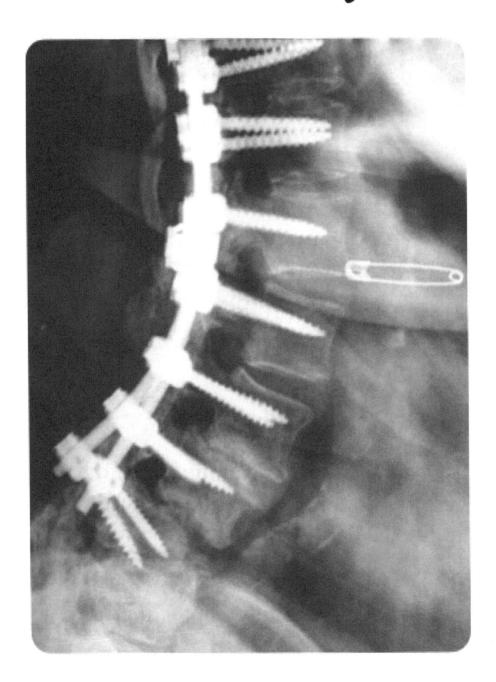

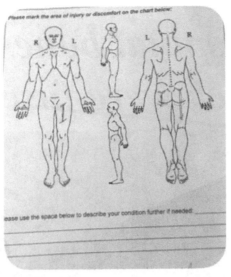

This pleasant woman has been coming to my office since 2014 off and on for back pain (see pain pattern above right).

In September of 2017, she said she fell and broke a bone in her low back. Since the fall, she has had two back surgeries.

I was blown away when I took her new X-ray and saw all the screws!

A year later, after 2 back surgeries, she can only sit for about 15 minutes, stand for 1 minute, and walk for 1 minute before she feels excruciating pain. Additionally, it hurts her to go from sitting to standing and anytime she coughs or sneezes.

It did not make sense to me as to why she had such a high number of fusions. Sadly, she did not know why either.

Seven spinal bones in her back were fused...

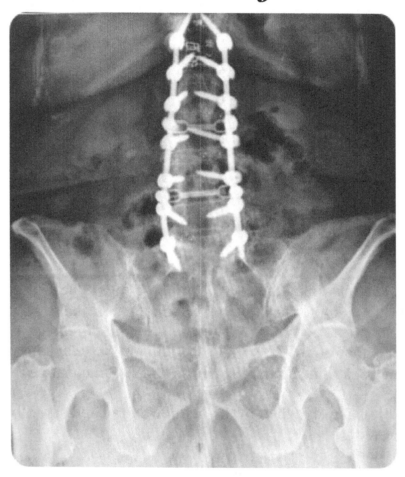

...and she is suffering more now, than ever before!

A 76-year-old female came to my office on a walker complaining of severe back pain, weakness in her legs and an occasional loss of bowel control.

She said that she had fusion surgery from a fall going up the steps in 2010.

Although the surgery helped get rid of her right leg pain, 8 years later she still suffers from debilitating back pain!

Neither her nor her husband knew why she had so many levels fused.

I did not accept her case.

Holy multi-level fusion!

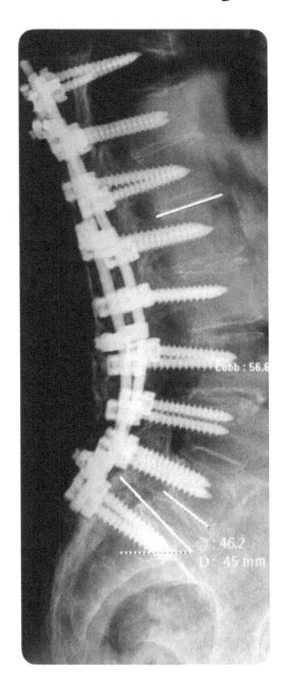

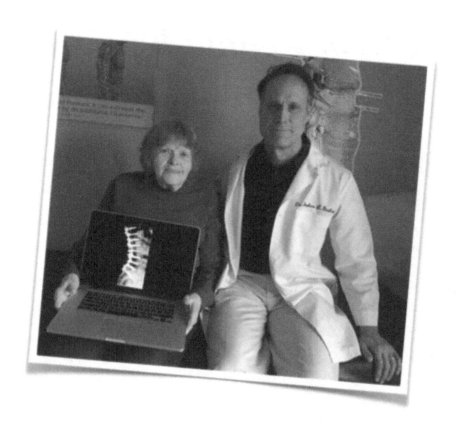

Jane came to me a few years ago and she could not stand or walk for more than a minute or two. She told me all she wanted to do was spend a day at the Horseshoe Casino without using a wheelchair.

She was on heavy doses of Hydrocodone, Gabapentin, and Cyclobenzaprine

I think this X-ray was <u>the biggest shocker in my 27 years of practice!</u>

"I wish I could have that moment back".

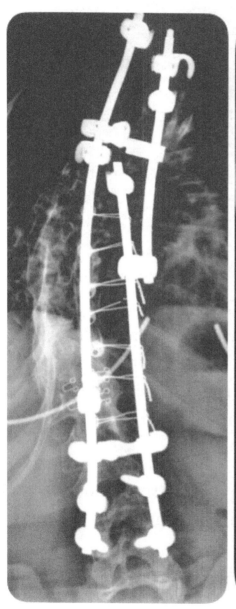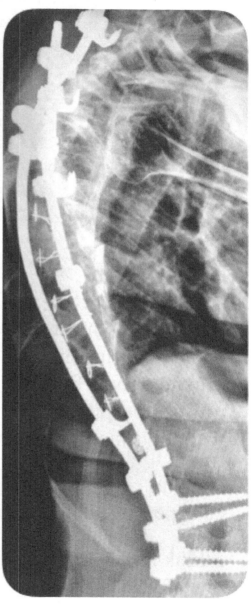

This 24-year-old woman came in my office right before this book was sent off for print. The x-ray was so compelling that I added it as the last x-ray of this chapter.

I did not treat this young lady, I just took this x-ray, as a part of her disability evaluation.

The only words I had with her were my x-ray instructions, telling her not to move or breathe.

I wish I had talked to her to have found out her story. I wish I could have that moment back.

EPILOGUE

Occam's Razor Principle

*Sometimes the questions are complicated
and the answers are simple.*
-Dr. Seuss

Years ago, I learned about the Occam's Razor Principle. This is a principle developed by William of Occam, an English Franciscan monk. He took his oath of poverty very seriously, meaning he just lived on what was only absolutely necessary, a form of simplicity.

His popular fame as a great logician rests on his maxim known as Occam's Razor. The term *razor* refers to distinguishing between two hypotheses by "shaving away" unnecessary assumptions. (1)

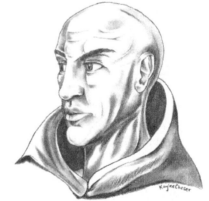

*William of
Occam*

His idea was, if there are two explanations for an occurrence, the simpler one is usually the right one! I have often found myself over the years applying this very same principle. When I am trying to make sense of something, I usually choose the simplest solution and when I exercise this judgement, not all the time, but most of the time, I have chosen correctly.

Occam's Razor applied to back pain

The 7 principles I have outlined that make for a strong, pain-free back: hydration, core, orthotics, walking, posture, mattresses and spinal adjustments, not only make sense, but they are simple.

Let me briefly run through a few of these steps, applying the "Occam's Razor" Principle.

- The arch in the right foot has fallen, causing the pelvis to drop on the same side, resulting in the spine pinching the nerve.

  Placing an orthotic in the shoe to raise the arch, to me, would seem like the simpler solution, compared to taking Gabapentin (a drug with many side effects), in an attempt to make the pain settle down.

- A weak core has caused the spine to sag, leading to back pain.

  Strengthening the core connects the dots easier for me than taking Meloxicam for extended periods of time.

- Finally, if an alignment problem is causing back and leg pain, adjusting the spine towards better alignment, seems like a simpler explanation and solution, than taking a month's supply of Baclofen.

Hopefully, you are getting the picture now!

Thank you for reading my book. Please share or recommend this book to a family member or friend, or both for that matter.

Chapter
Summaries

Introduction
Spinal Fusions

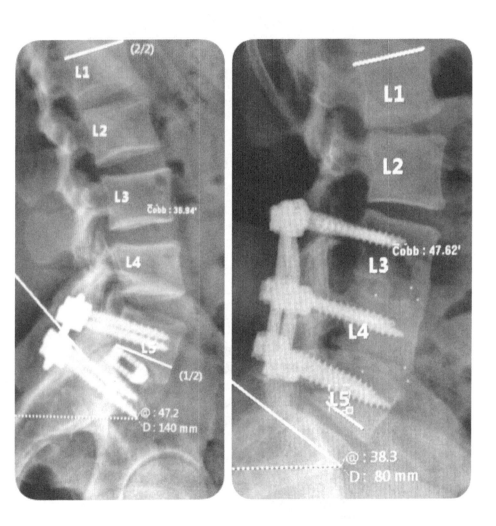

Single Level Fusion   **Two Level Fusion**

Multi-Level Fusion

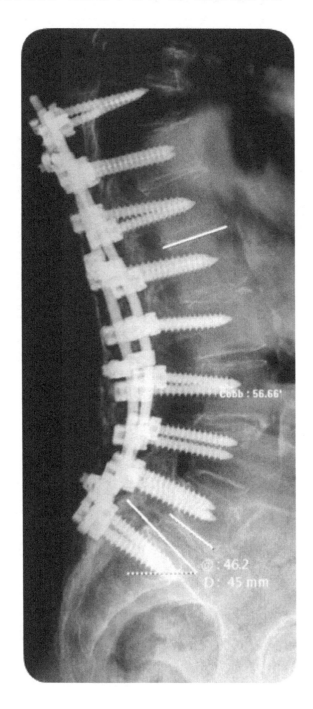

Adjacent segment disease

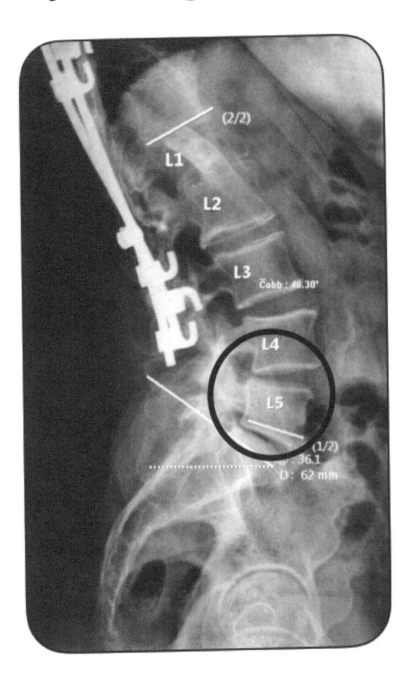

<u>Facts About Back Pain</u> (7)

- **8 out of 10 will experience back problems at some point in their life.**

- **Back problems are more common in women (30.2) than men (26.4).**

- **The majority of back pain comes from desk workers: 54%**

- **More than one in three adults say back pain impacts their everyday activities, including sleep.**

- **$50,000,000,000 of treatments in 2016.**

- **$100,000,000,000 of indirect costs in 2016.**

The Beginnings
Our Framework

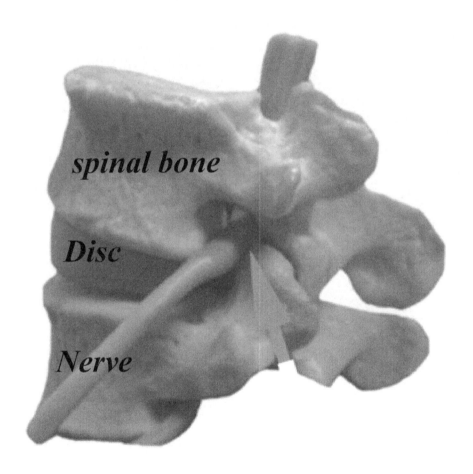

spinal bone

Disc

Nerve

Spinal X-ray
Normal Alignment

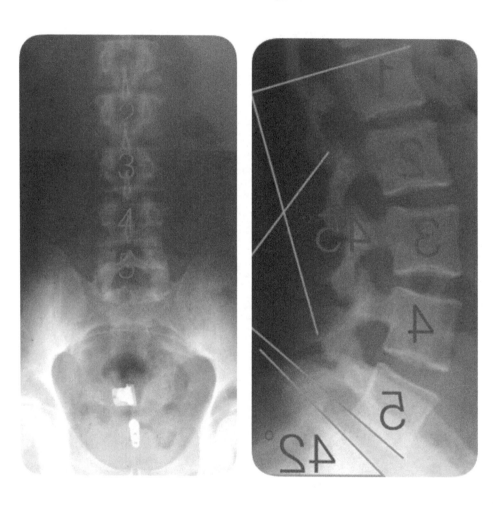

Front   **Side**

MRI

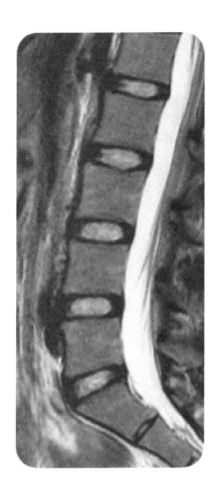 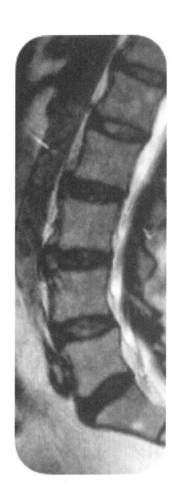

Normal
White discs
Strong

Dried Up Discs
Black discs
Weaker-may collapse

Discs

Normal-
Jelly in the middle

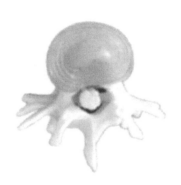

Bulging -
*Jelly pushes
the disc back*

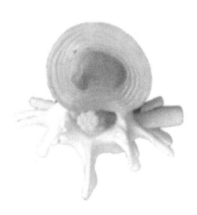

Herniated -
*Jelly comes
out of disc*

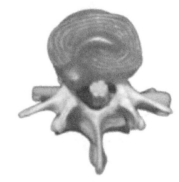

MRI-
Bulging and Herniated discs

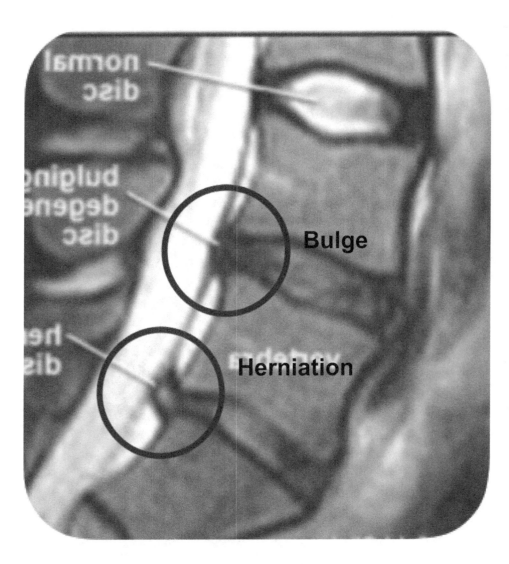

Bulge

Herniation

MRI-
Collapsed disc

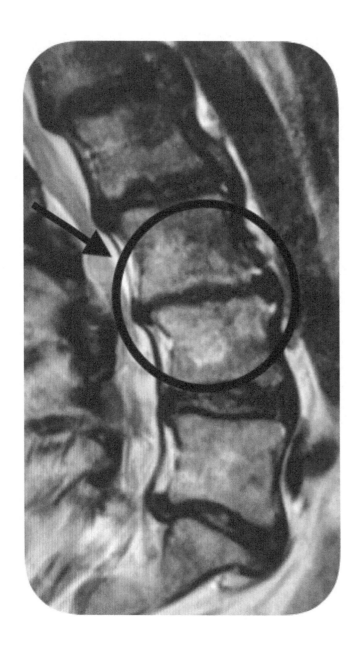

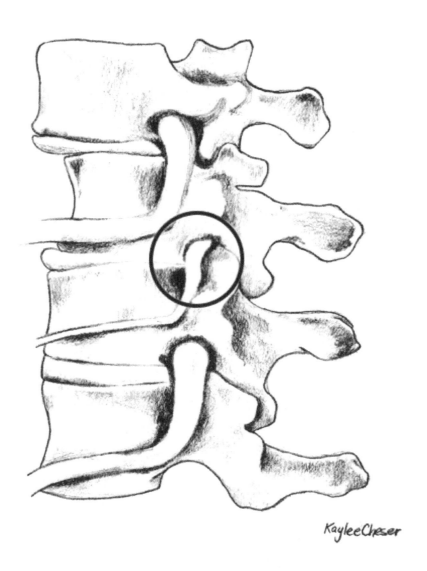

Pinched Nerve

Tips for a healthy disc:

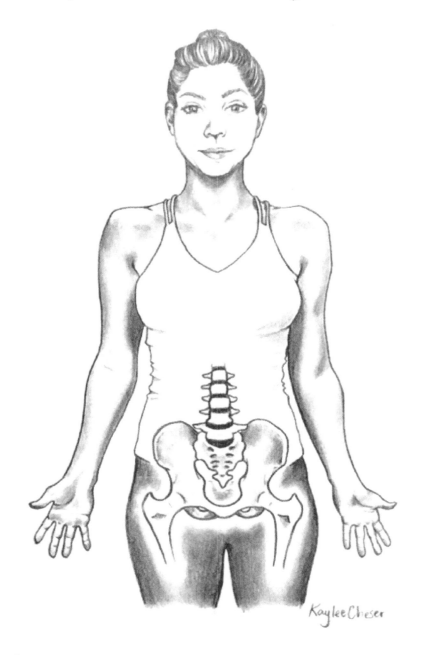

✓ **Keep the spine in good alignment**

✓ *Exercise*

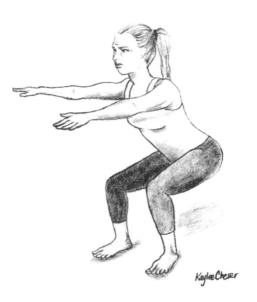

✓ *Hydrate Well*

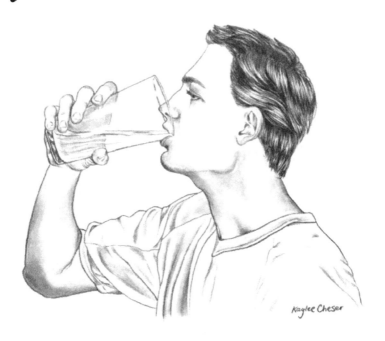

✓ *Rest*

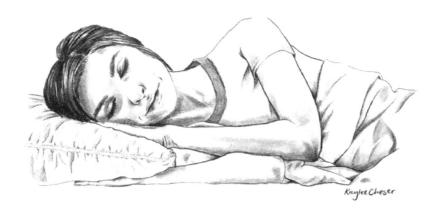

✓ *Weight reduction*

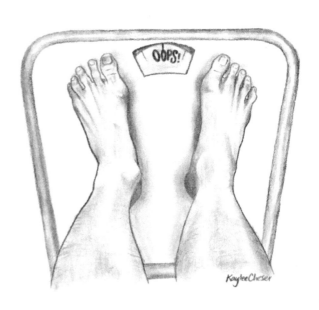

STEP 1
Hydration

$$\frac{Body\ Weight}{2} = \text{ounces of hydration per day}$$

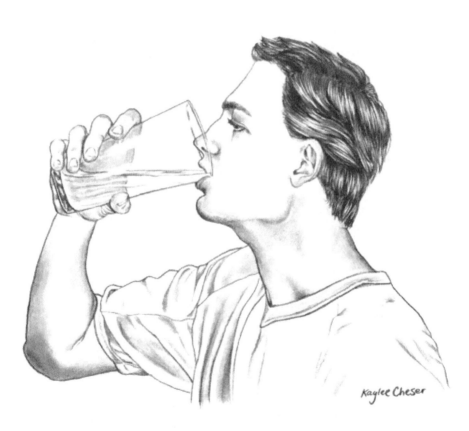

Kaylee Cheser

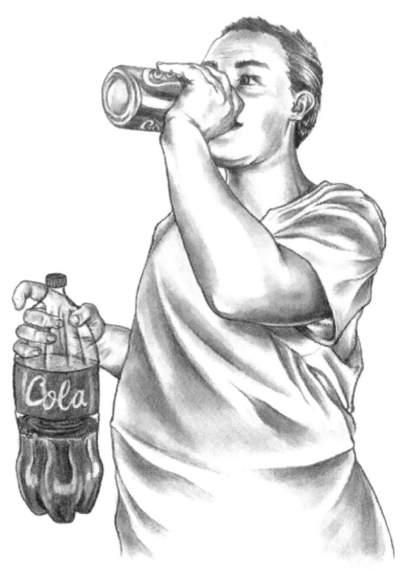

Kaylee Cheser

Soft drinks and caffeine products dehydrate the disc!

Imbibition: the water we drink is pumped into the disc for re-hydration as long as there is plenty of it in our body

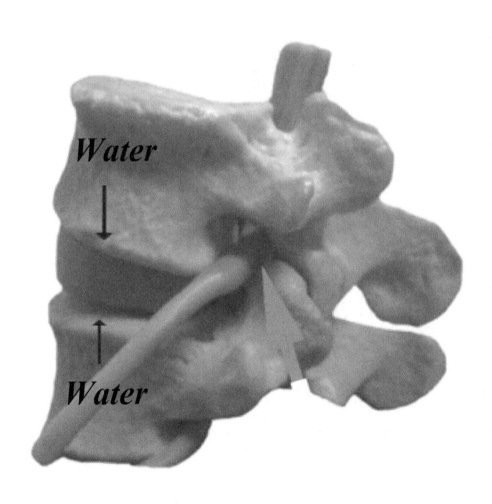

Water

Water

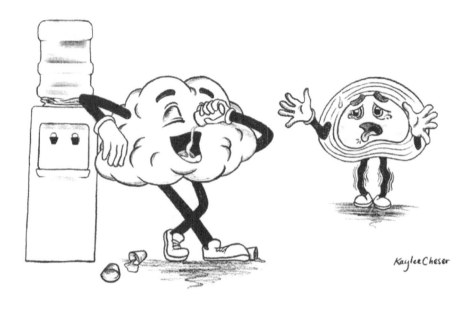

The brain, cardiovascular system and lungs get first dibs on the water you ingest, while the ligaments and discs are in the back of the line!

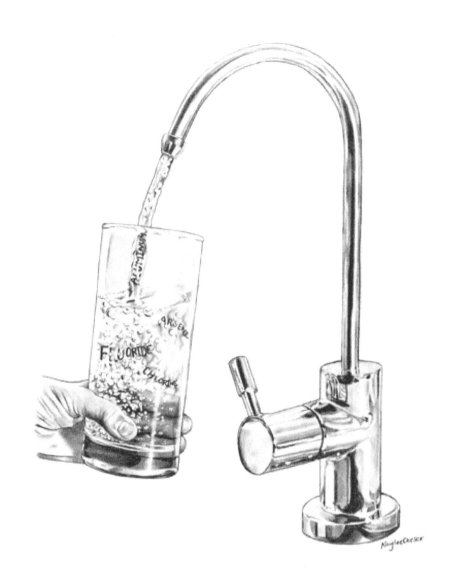

There are dangerous chemicals in tap water!

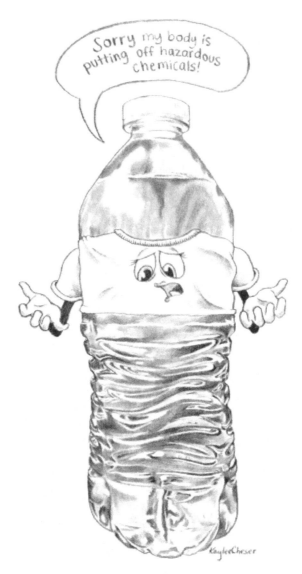

Plastic water bottles put off dangerous chemicals!

Home Water Purifiers

Berkey Water Filter System

$228

Amazon.com

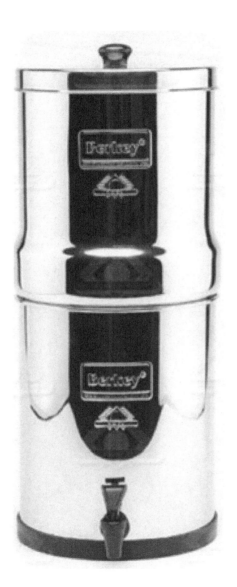

STEP 2
Core

Muscles-front and side

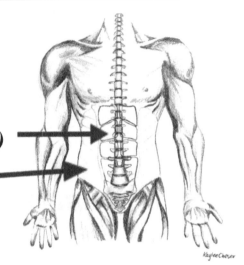

Mid core
(Rectus Abdominus)

Side Core
(Obliques)

Core Muscles-Back

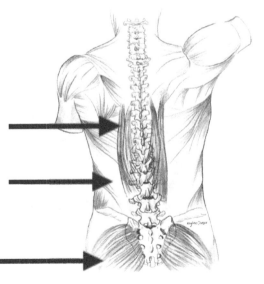

Erector Spinae

Quadratus Lumborum

Gluteus Maximus

Easy Core Exercises:

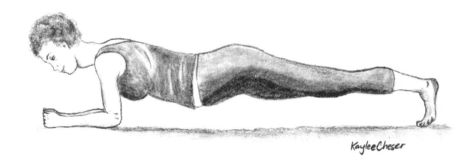

Planks

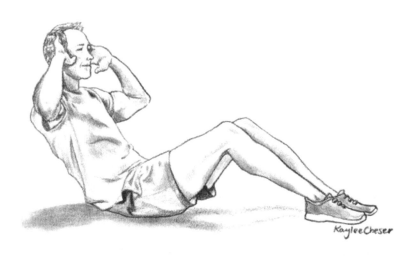

Abdominal Crunches

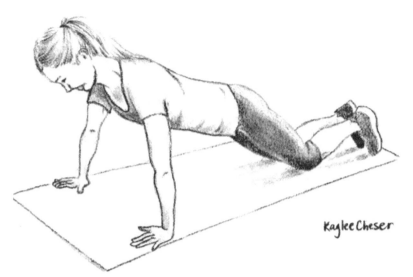

Kaylee Cheser

Push ups

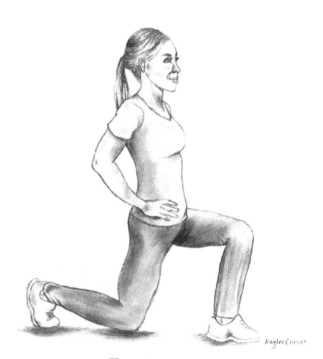

Kaylee Cheser

Lunges

One armed
dumbbells

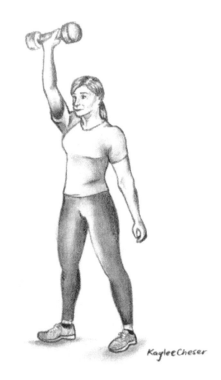

KayleeCheser

Wall

Push-Ups

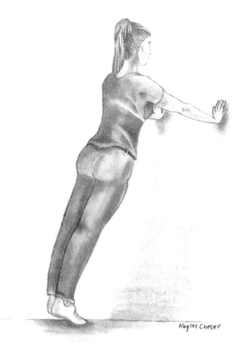

KayleeCheser

Air
Squats

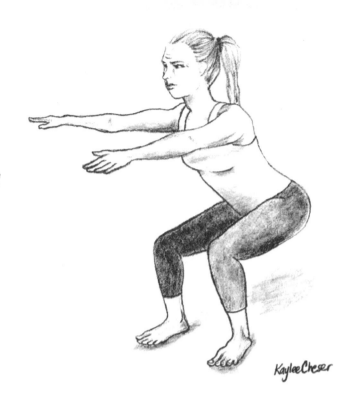

Warrior
Pose

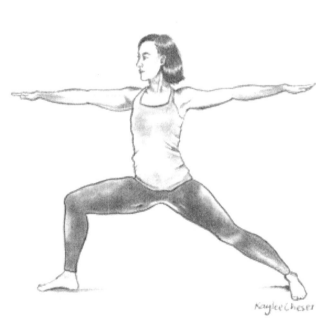

STEP 3
Orthotics

Good arches

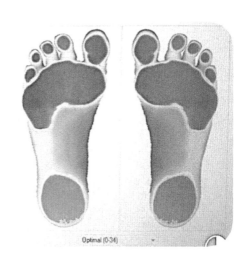

Optimal (0-34)

Bad arches

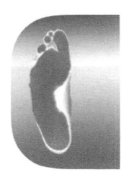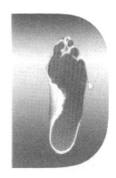

Whole Body Alignment

Straight Man

Crooked Man

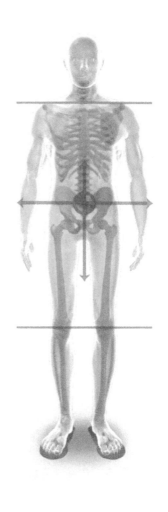

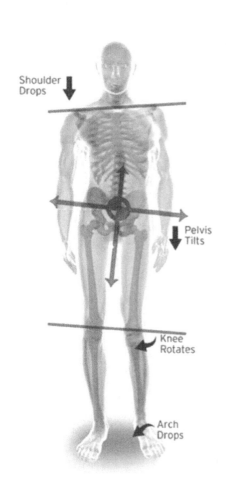

Good Arch
Good Alignment

Dropped Arch
Bad Alignment

Custom Orthotics

Foot Levelers

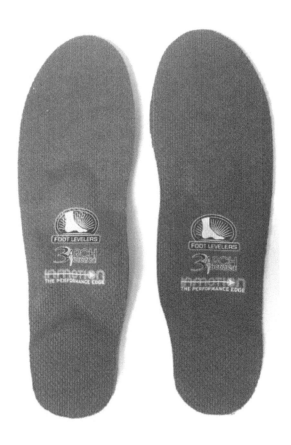

The "3-Arch" orthotic
Dr. Graham's Favorite

Price: $295

STEP 4
Walking

Dr. Graham's Favorite Fitbit

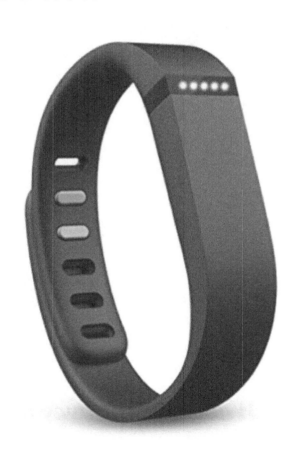

Fitbit Flex
$49.99 at Target

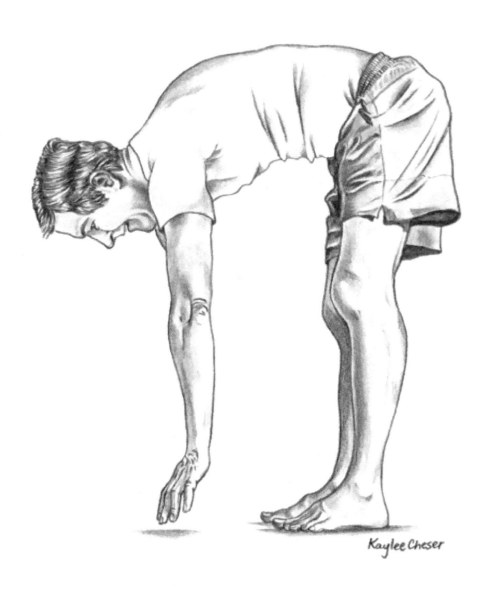

Walking improves flexibility

Walking Shoes

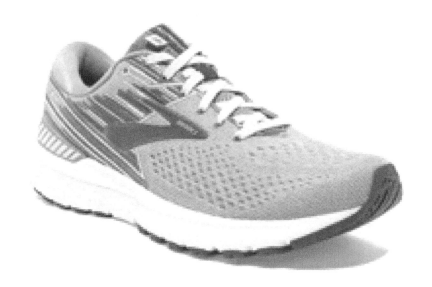

Dr. Graham's favorite shoe
Brooks Adrenaline GTS 19
$130

STEP 5
Posture

Intra-discal Pressures: lowest to highest

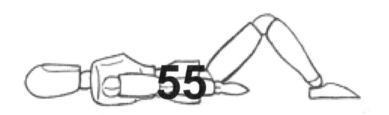

Laying down
Lowest Disc Pressure

Standing

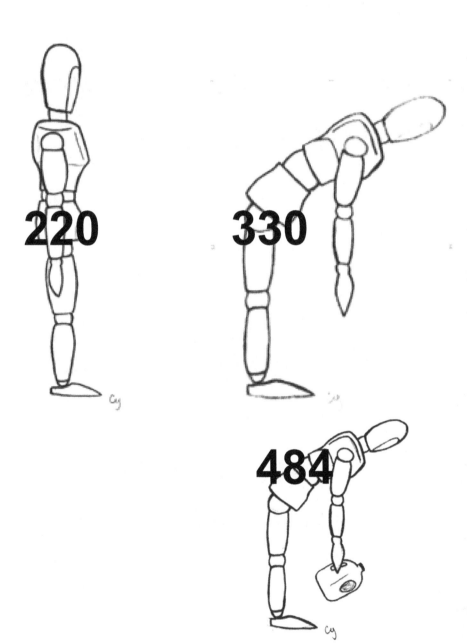

220

330

484

Sitting
Highest Disc Pressure

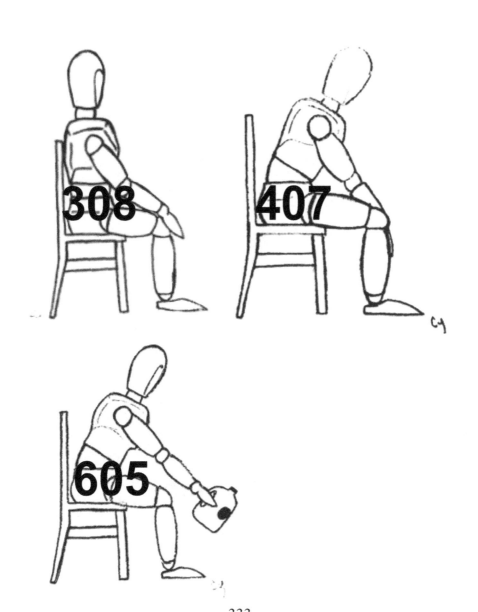

Postural Exercises

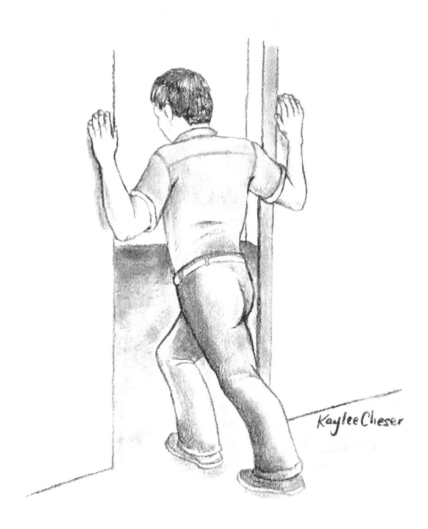

Pec Stretch

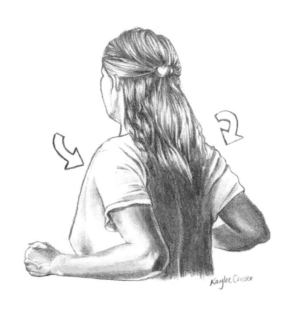

Shoulder blade pinches

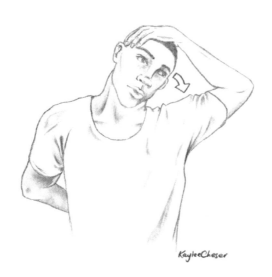

Trap Stretch
(Trap=Trapezius muscle)

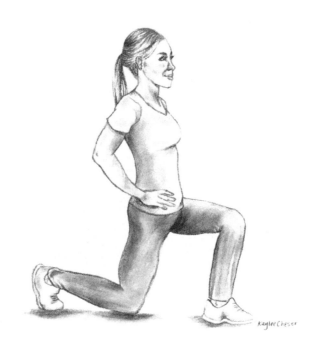

Hip Flexor Stretch

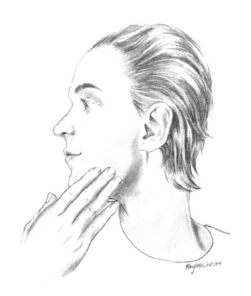

Neck Stretches

Postural Work Station Aids

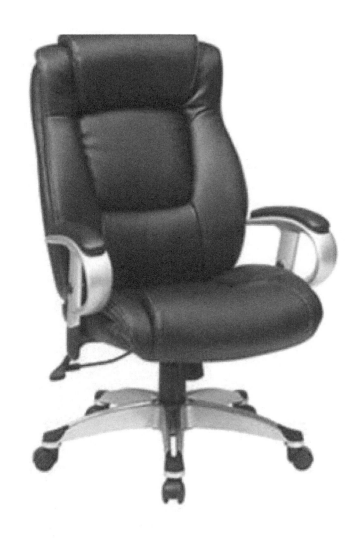

Adjustable Chair
$195-Office Depot

Exercise
Ball

$50
Amazon.com

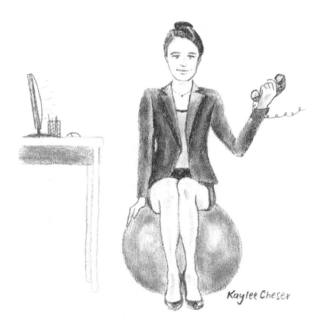

Kaylee Cheser

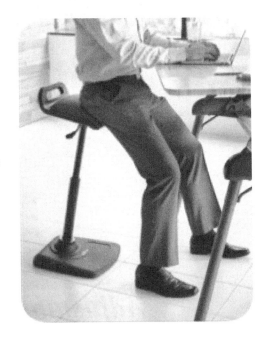

VERICHAIR

$195

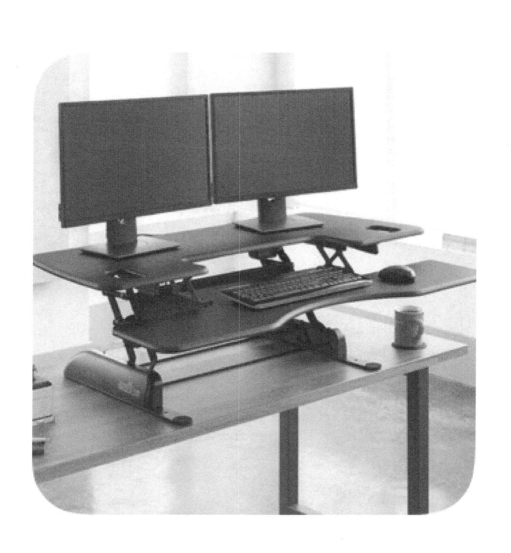

VARIDESK

$395

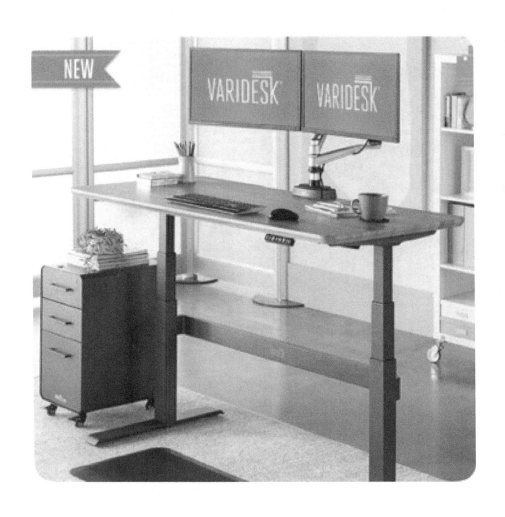

VARIDESK
ProDesk 60
$995

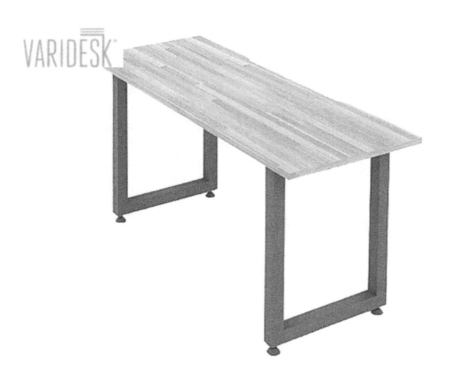

Butcher Block

VARIDESK

$399

Great Posture at the Desk

Relax-A-Bac
Lumbar Cushion
$25
Amazon.com

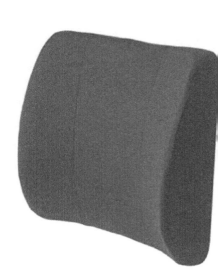

Great Posture in the Car

Dreamer Car Auto Seat Lumbar Support

$33.49

Amazon.com

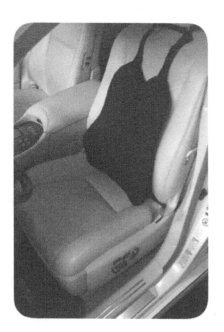

Posture Corrector

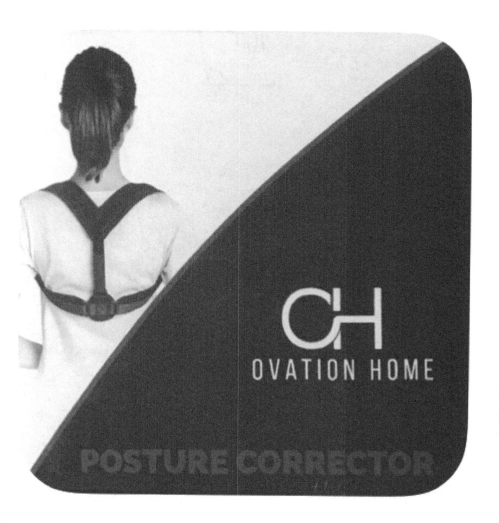

$21 Amazon.com

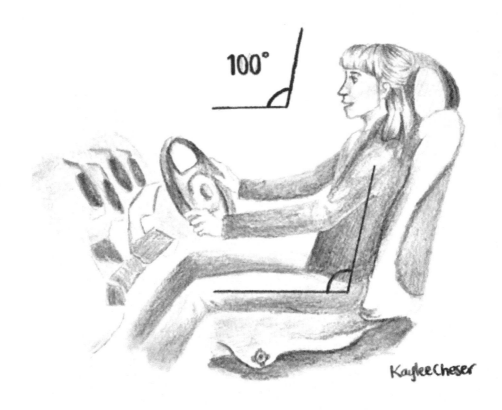

Good posture in the Car

STEP 6
Mattresses

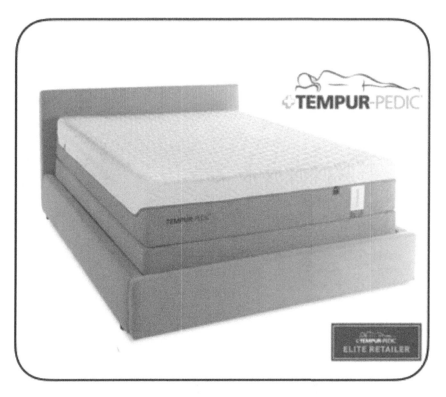

Best Mattress for comfort and spinal alignment.

"Anyone who owns a spine, should own a Tempur-Pedic!"

-Stephen Graham, D.C.

Pillows

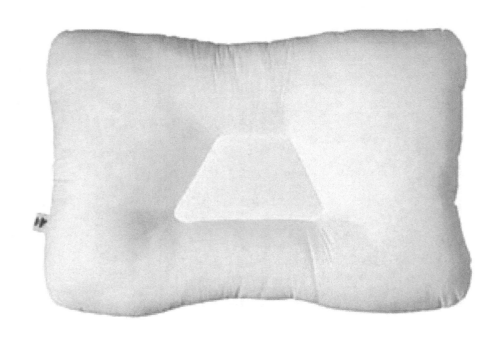

Best Pillow

Tri-Core Pillow
$50 Amazon.com

STEP 7
Spinal Adjustments

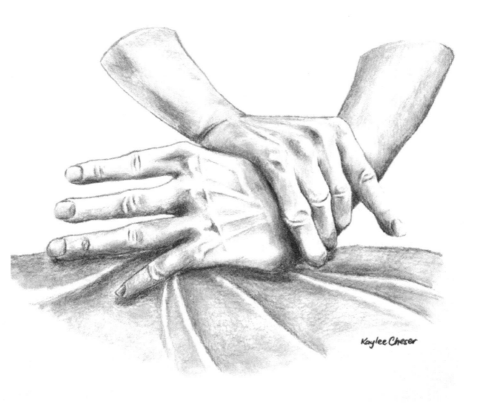

Kaylee Cheser

Pinched nerve caused by a compressed, misaligned spine.

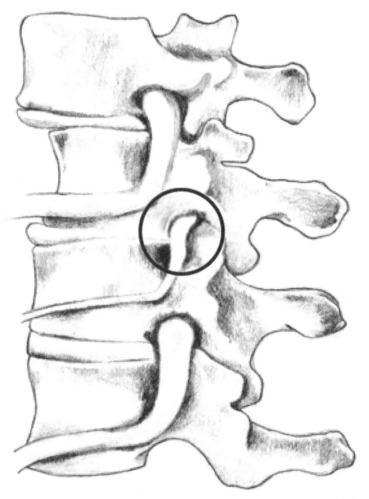

KayleeCheser

Correcting a pinched nerve by de-compressing and re-aligning spine.

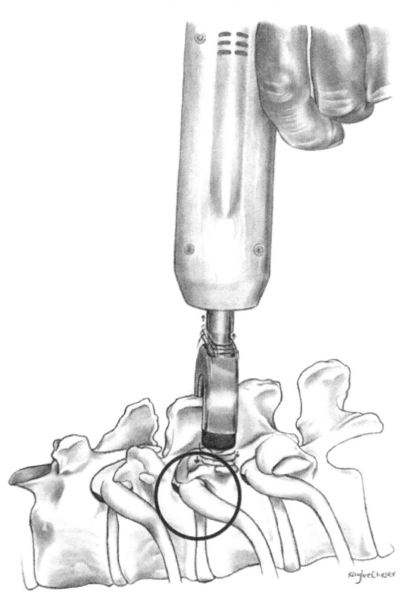

ABOUT THE AUTHOR

Dr. Stephen Graham is a practicing chiropractor of 27 years. He attended Logan College of Chiropractic from 1985-1989. After completing his internship, passing his national and state boards, and completing a residency program, he came back to Louisville to practice. He had always wanted to return to his home roots because he was born, reared, and attended school there (St. Albert the Great, Trinity, and Bellarmine College).

Because of his own personal history, he has a real passion for correcting back pain and especially sympathetic towards those people who are struggling with back-related health issues. That is the very reason that most of his post graduate conferences revolve around the latest treatment techniques for back pain.

Dr. Graham is married to Donna, who is from New Albany, Indiana and they have a dog named Samson. They attend Southeast Christian Church in Louisville.

ABOUT THE ILLUSTRATOR

Kaylee Cheser is a resident of Louisville, Kentucky. She is a graduate of Eastern High School where she received numerous awards from the art department. In her time there, she was a part of the Vans Custom Culture Team for two years. They competed nationwide and finished as a top five in the country.

She contracts out for commission work and creates and sells her personal artwork as well.

Footnotes

Introduction

1. "Degenerative Disc Disease". *University of Maryland Medical Center.* Retrieved 2017-01-04

2. www.biographyonline.net, *Top 10 Inventors.*

BEGINNINGS

1. Washington Post, *Rise in Spinal Fusion Surgeries May Be Driven Partly by Financial Incentives, Study Says*, Peter Whoriskey, November 13, 2013.

2. US Population by <u>year-multpl.com</u>

3. Washington Post, *Rise in Spinal Fusion Surgeries May Be Driven Partly by Financial Incentives, Study Says*, Peter Whoriskey, November 13, 2013.

4. www.aca. *Alarming Escalation of Fusion Surgery – What Can be Done?,* Ron Feise, DC/Thursday, January 07, 2016

5. www.laserspinesurgery.com, *What causes failed back surgery syndrome?*

6. www.laserspinesurgery.com, *What causes failed back surgery syndrome?*

7. www.acatoday.org/patients/Health-Wellness-Information/Back-Pain-Facts-and-Statistics

8. <u>www.Gamesparks.com</u>, 100 Billion Dollars.

9.www.medicine.com, *Tylenol Liver Damage: Signs, Symptoms, Dosage,*

10. www.kidney.org, *Watch out for Your Kidneys When You Use Medicines for Pain ...*

11. YourNewsWire.com,100,000 Deaths Per Year In The U.S. Caused By Prescription Drugs, February 6, 2015, Jacqui Deevoy

12. Web MD, What are the side effects of steroid injections?

STEP 1

1. CatholicCulture.org, The Day the Mass Changed, How it Happened and Why -- Part I, Susan Benofy

2. Wikipedia, Intervertebral disc -

3. Medical News Today, All About the Central Nervous System,Last updated Fri 22 December 2017, Seunggu Han, MD

4. Hong CH, Park JS, Jung KJ and Kim WJ. Measurement of the normal lumbar intervertebral disc space using magnetic resonance imaging. Asian Spine J 2010; 4: 1-6.

5. Urban, Jill PG; Roberts, Sally (2003-03-11). "Degeneration of the intervertebral disc". *Arthritis Res Ther.* 5: 120

6. www.healthline.com/human-body-maps/intervertebral-disk

7. 10 Symptoms of Spinal Stenosis - RM Healthy rmhealthy.com/10-symptoms-spinal-stenosis

8. Wikipedia, Degenerative disc disease

9. Laser Spine Institute, Bulging disc causes

10. MayoClinic.org, herniated disc

11. www.spineuniverse.com, Lumbar herniated disc-risk factors

12. BackPainRelief.net, What Is a Collapsed Disc?

13. www.rmhealthy.com, *10 Symptoms of Spinal Stenosis*

14. LaserSpineInstitute.com, *Degeneration causes*

15. Wikihow.com, *How to do anything, Improving Back and Bone Health.*

16. CancerFightingStrategies.*com pH and Cancer Acidic pH Levels Can Lead To Cancer...Normalizing pH Can Stop Cancer In Its Tracks*

17. www.spinehealth.com,*Controlling Degenerative Disc Disease-Three Things You Can Do.*

18. www.nhs.uk/Conditions/Slipped-disc/Pages/Treatment

19.www.choosemyplate.gov/fruits-tips

20. thepainsource.com, *Intradiscal Pressures in Various Everyday positions and Activities*, Azian Tariq, D.O., August 21,2010

21. www.eldoamethod.com, *Heal your Back Pain With Eldoa and Water.*, Stephanie McCusker, October 27, 2015.

STEP 2

1. www.clinical gate.com, The Intervertebral Disc: Normal, Aging, and Pathologic, Edward Westrick, MD, Gwendolyn Sowa, MD, PhD, James D. Kang, MD

2. www.undergroundhealthreporter.com, Fact or Myth: Are You Taller in the Morning?

3. H.H. Mitchell, Journal of Biological Chemistry 158

4. www.Dr.Mercola.com, "How drinking pure water can improve every facet of your health"

STEP 3

1. Journal of Spinal Disorders and Technique, *The Stabilizing System of the Spine. Part I. Function, Dysfunction, Adaptation and Enhancement*, Manohar M. Panjabi, August 1992.

2. Human Kinetics, *Core Assessment and Training*, Jason Brumitt, MSPT.

3. Wikipedia, *Core (anatomy)*.

4. Harvard Health Publications. *"The real-world benefits of strengthening your core"* (2012).

5. TravelStrong.net, *7 of the Best Core Exercises (You can do anywhere)*.

6. HealthHarvard.edu, *The Real World Benefit of strengthening Your Core*.

7. www.riversidekettlebells.com, *10-benefits-of-kettlebell Training*

STEP 4

1. Footlevelers.com, *Arch Collapse*

2. WebMD, *What are Fallen Arches?*

3. WebMD, *What are Fallen Arches?*

4. Footlevelers.com, *Plantar Fasciitis*

5. Footlevelers.com, *The 5 Red Flags of Pronation*

STEP 5

1. WebMd.com, *10 Ways to Manage Low Back Pain at Home.*

2. Mercola.com, *How Walking Benefits Your Health and Longevity*

3. Breakingmuscle.com, *Forget Crunches: How to Actually Strengthen Your Core*, Andrew Read.

4. P.W. Hodges, A.E.M. Eriksson, D. Shirley, S.C. Gandevia. *'Lumbar Spine Stiffness is Increased by Intra-Abdominal Pressure'*

5. Livestrong.com, Can Walking Improve Circulation?, Sharon Perkins.

6. Stretchcoach.com, *Walking Stretching Exercises*. Brad Walker, January 18, 2009

7. Osteopenia3.com, *Is Walking: a good bone density exercise or what?*

8. Fitday.com, *Understanding Weight Loss: How to Lose 20 Pounds By Walking*

STEP 6

1, 2, 3, 4, 5,. thepainsource.com, *Intradiscal Pressures in Various Everyday positions and Activities*, Azian Tariq, D.O., August 21,2010

6. American Physical Therapy Association (2012) *Most Americans ....Live with Low Back Pain – and Don't Seek Treatment.*

7. www.sciencedirect.com, *Internal Oblique and Transversus Abdominis Muscle Fatigue*

8. thepainsource.com, *Intradiscal Pressures in Various Everyday positions and Activities*, Azian Tariq, D.O., August 21,2010.

STEP 7

1. med.harvard.edu, *Changes in Sleep with Age*. Dr. Richard Ferber, December 2007.

2, 3, 4, 5 positivehealth.com, *How Sleep Surfaces Affect Our Back*, Bill Ancell, January 2000.

BONUS MATERIAL I

1. SoutheasternSpineInstitute.com, *Does Health Insurance Cover Back Surgery?*

2. Spine-health.com, *Spinal Fusion Surgery Recovery: One to Three Months Post-Operation*, John E. Sherman, M.D.

3. Spine-health.com, *TLIF Back Surgery Success Rates and Risk,* Stephen P. Montgomery, M.D.

EPILOGUE

1. Wikipedia, William of Ockham

Notes:

Notes:

Made in the USA
Middletown, DE
15 September 2019